MENOPAUSE

Dr Sandra Cabot, M.B.B.S.,D.R.C.O.G., is a well known media doctor and author of the best selling books: *Women's Health, Don't Let Your Hormones Ruin Your Life, The Body Shaping Diet.*

Sandra is a consultant to the Australian Women's Health Advisory Service, has regularly appeared on many national TV shows, including the Ray Martin Midday Show, had her own talk back show on radio 2GB for two years, writes for *Woman's Day* and is a much sought after public speaker on women's health. She has extensive clinical experience in women's health, hormonal disorders and naturopathic medicine.

Sandra is sometimes known as the 'flying doctor' as she frequently flies herself to many of Australia's country towns to hold health forums for rural women. These help to raise funds for local women's refuges and women's health services. She spent considerable time working in the Department of Obstetrics and Gynaecology in a large missionary hospital in the Himalayan foothills of India.

Sandra has communicated with women via TV and radio and receives thousands of letters from women all over Australia. Thus she is acutely aware of the health problems and needs of women from many different backgrounds.

MENOPAUSE

DR SANDRA CABOT MD

HORMONE REPLACEMENT THERAPY
and its
NATURAL ALTERNATIVES

First published 1991 by Women's Health Advisory Service
155 Eagle Creek Rd, Werombi 2570, NSW, Australia (046) 531 445
Reprinted 1991 (twice), 1993, 1994.

Cabot, Sandra
    Menopause
    Bibliography
    Includes index
    ISBN 0 646 03768 4
    1. Menopause—Popular works. 2. Middle Aged Women—
    Health and hygiene
    1. Women's Health Advisory Service (NSW) II Title
    (Series: Cabot, Sandra—Women's Health Guides For Life)

Printed and bound in Australia by
Australian Print Group, Melbourne Australia.

CONTENTS

ACKNOWLEDGEMENTS

I would like to acknowledge the professional
and creative assistance of my two editors
Diane Blackwell and Stephanie Lewis who
enabled me to put scientific breakthroughs into
everyday language. Without their faith and
support this book would not have been so special.
I would also like to thank Lydia Sharan for her
superb typing skills, her dedication and
generosity of spirit.

FOREWORD

by Dr Valentine Vargassoff M.B.B.S.,F.R.A.C.P.,F.R.C.P.A.

Sadly, many women still remain confused, bewildered and out of touch with the tremendous advances in hormonal therapy.

Finally we have a well researched, easy to read, warm and relatable handbook that puts all of the information in a nutshell. Not surprisingly, it has taken a woman doctor, who knows how it feels herself and through her experience with thousands of patients, to awaken women to the tremendous potential of hormone replacement therapy and preventative medicine.

Menopause: Hormone Replacement Therapy and its Natural Alternatives is useful for women of all ages who want to make the time of midlife and beyond a positive and healthy experience. I can thoroughly recommend this book for those wanting to keep pace with the evolution of women during the next decade of the 20th century.

Dr Valentine Vargassoff is a Sydney physician and pathologist who specialises in the menopause and breast disorders.

The information contained in this book is intended to be a general guide for menopausal women. Neither Dr. Sandra Cabot or the publisher can accept responsibility for your health, nor any side effects of treatments described in this book. You should always be guided by your own doctor and remain under his or her supervision, when following any of the treatments (even naturopathic) in this book.

INTRODUCTION

The terms "menopause" and "change of life" often arouse feelings of fear, dread, uncertainty and confusion and although the menopause is the greatest physical milestone in a woman's life it does not have to be traumatic or painful.

This book is your menopause handbook and serves as a lifeline to guide you through this often awesome and bewildering time of life. It discusses all your options in a simple and clear way.

Around the age of 50 years the biological clock stops ticking, signalling the loss of fertility and the loss of the female sex hormones oestrogen and progesterone.

Vitally important questions are raised by the loss of these parts of our feminine identity. Questions such as:

How will I feel mentally, physically and sexually without the female sex hormones?

Will I age more rapidly without oestrogen in my body?

Will I still be able to function and compete efficiently with younger women in the work place?

Will my husband lose interest in me and take a younger lover?

Will I lose my femininity and look more masculine?

If I have a premature menopause can I still have a baby?

What are my risks for osteoporosis?

Read on and all these questions and many more will be answered.

A woman passing through the menopause and beyond needs to know all her options. For example:

Do I need to take female hormones in the form of hormone replacement therapy?

Can I have natural hormone replacement therapy instead of the old fashioned synthetic hormones? If one type of hormone replacement therapy does not help me, can I take it in other forms?

What is the difference between hormone pills, injections, patches, creams, implants or pessaries?

If I don't want hormone replacement therapy what natural supplements can help me to cope with the menopause?

What type of diet and nutritional supplements should I take to slow down the ageing process?

Remember you can master the symptoms of your menopause and emerge with your vitality, femininity, sexuality and peace of mind intact. Indeed in many cases the change of life can be a change for the better.

This book is dedicated to my two magnificent
sisters Madeleine and Paula.
And to all the women of the world whose
health we have an obligation to insure.

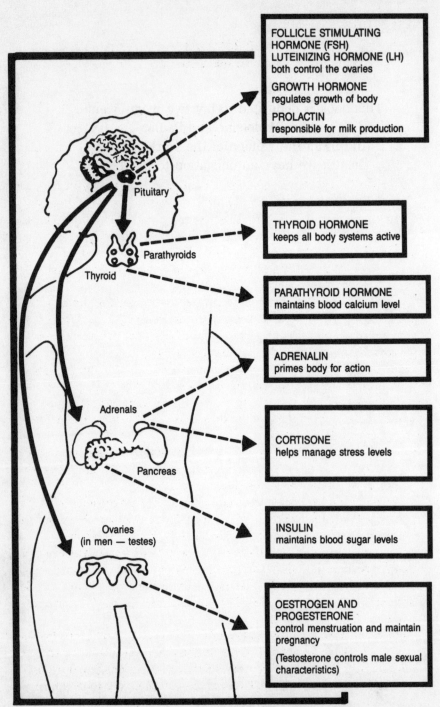

FOLLICLE STIMULATING
HORMONE (FSH)
LUTEINIZING HORMONE (LH)
both control the ovaries

GROWTH HORMONE
regulates growth of body

PROLACTIN
responsible for milk production

THYROID HORMONE
keeps all body systems active

PARATHYROID HORMONE
maintains blood calcium level

ADRENALIN
primes body for action

CORTISONE
helps manage stress levels

INSULIN
maintains blood sugar levels

OESTROGEN AND
PROGESTERONE
control menstruation and maintain
pregnancy

(Testosterone controls male sexual
characteristics)

Pituitary

Parathyroids

Thyroid

Adrenals

Pancreas

Ovaries
(in men — testes)

ENDOCRINE GLANDS AND THEIR HORMONES– DIAGRAM 1

CHAPTER 1

WHAT IS A HORMONE?

Before we deal with the menopause in depth it is important for you to understand what a hormone is and how it functions in your body. Hormones are body chemicals that carry messages from one part of the body to another. They are made in specialised glands located in various places in our body and are circulated in the blood to body cells where they make their presence dramatically felt. These specialised glands are called endocrine glands (see diagram 1.)

The thyroid gland manufactures thyroid hormone, the adrenal glands manufacture adrenalin and cortisone and the ovaries produce the sex hormones oestrogen and progesterone, to name a few of the many hormones required to keep our cells functioning in harmony.

Compared to our nervous system, hormones tend to act more slowly as they are concerned with controlling the chemistry of cells. Hormones determine the rate at which our cells burn up food substances and release energy and whether our cells should produce milk, hair, secretions, enzymes or some other metabolic product.

Hormones are extremely potent molecules and in some cases less than a millionth of a gram is sufficient to exert their effects. They are far too small to be seen even under a microscope.

After they have completed their tasks, hormones are broken down by the cells themselves or are carried to the liver for breakdown. They are then excreted or used again to manufacture new hormone molecules.

Hormones can be likened to chemical keys that turn vitally important metabolic locks in our cells. The turning of these locks stimulates activity within the cells of our brain, intestines, muscles, genital organs and skin. Indeed all our cells are influenced to some degree by these amazing hormonal keys. (See Diagram 2).

Without the hormonal keys the metabolic locks on our cells remain closed and the full potential of our cells is not realised. Imagine a corporation where the employees are unable to communicate with the managing director and are left to do their own thing. The corporation lacks any unified direction or growth. This chaos is what happens in your cells without hormones.

13

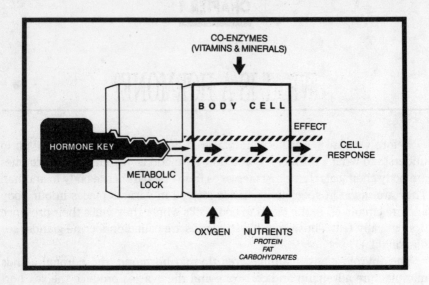

DIAGRAM 2

CHAPTER 2

CAN HORMONES RUIN YOUR LIFE?

An imbalance or lack of hormones can shatter your life. Hormones are vital to make you sexually responsive, passionate, sensitive and to sustain mental drive.

According to consultant gynaecologist John Studd of the Menopause Clinic at Kings College Hospital, London, adequate amounts of the female sex hormones keep women "out of the orthopaedic wards, the divorce courts and the madhouse". Before Hormone Replacement Therapy (HRT) became available, a significant percentage of menopausal women suffered a severe mid-life crisis which was called in medical terminology "involutional melancholia". This old fashioned term describes the total shrinkage of the mind and body that could occur without the presence of the sex hormones. Some of these women became so profoundly depressed that they were institutionalised for the rest of their lives.

Hormones control many aspects of human behaviour and emotions and help to make you a mentally competent functional person. They are involved in the system of psycho-neuro-endocrinology which is the complex interaction of the mind, nerves and hormonal (endocrine) system. We are only beginning to understand that many mental illnesses such as manic depression and schizophrenia have a chemical basis.

The brain's own natural "happy hormones" act on the pleasure centres in the brain and help us cope with pain and emotional turmoil. If these brain hormones, the endorphins, serotonin and biogenic amines become depleted, we may suffer with a deep and gloomy depressive illness.

Imbalances of various hormones can create devastating and insidious signs of malfunction and suffering such as personality changes, panic attacks, agoraphobia, poor memory, insomnia, frigidity, loss of sexuality, obesity, blood sugar problems, allergies, inflammation and this list is far from exhaustive.

The medical speciality of the treatment of hormonal disorders is called endocrinology. We can now measure accurately with blood tests the levels of the vast majority of the body's hormones. We are able to **replace** these hormones if the various glands of the endocrine system fail to manufacture

15

adequate amounts of their specialised hormones. This is how the term "hormone replacement therapy" (HRT) came to be.

Hormones — yes they can make you or break you, make your life heaven or hell and be responsible for untold miseries. Thanks to modern-day bio-technology, genetic engineering, pharmacology and nutritional medicine, we can now control our hormones. This is truly powerful medicine with implications as momentous as the atomic bomb.

In this book you will discover the influence of hormones upon your mental and emotional state, your ability to succeed, your sexuality and appearance, and the rate at which you will age. You will be amazed by the way hormones influence your menstrual cycle, immune system, and your chances of getting osteoporosis, cancer and cardiovascular disease.

The questions answered throughout this book are those most asked by my women patients in the surgery.

CHAPTER 3

HOW ATTITUDES HAVE CHANGED

My fifty-four year old patient who had sat for hours on the bus all the way from Lightning Ridge to seek help, flopped into the chair on the other side of my desk with a desperate and exhausted look in her eyes. She told me that male doctors had no time to listen to her woes and merely threw their arms up in the air, saying that she was getting on in years. She said that life was cruel for women going through the menopause and that she felt like a sexless, emotionless "it". Indeed, she felt as if she had been cheated by life and did not want to hear "That's life, it's just part of getting on in years."

I have heard countless tales like this and perhaps because I am a woman and not just a doctor, I can empathise with the plight of many frustrated women like the one from Lightning Ridge who do not want to be a victim of a deficiency of female hormones.

We do not have to suffer this problem in loneliness and isolation as there are real, safe and simple solutions for today's menopausal woman, solutions to revitalise and rekindle our former mental and physical wellbeing and slow down the ravages of time upon our minds and bodies. We are all in the same boat, so to speak, united by the inevitable and irrevocable fact that our ovaries have a limited lifespan. However, every woman is a beautiful individual and may need a special or unique programme of Hormone Replacement Therapy (HRT), counselling, nutritional supplements, dietary modification and general medical treatment to ensure that she finds the passage to midlife and beyond a fruitful and pleasant voyage. Occasionally, women are still being told that the menopause is part of mother nature and should be accepted as our mothers had gracefully accepted it. In fact, our mothers may have died and still die today from some of the long-term complications of the menopause.

The attitude of doctors towards menopausal women has changed slowly over the last century. In the year 1850, the most famous gynaecologist of the day, a Frenchman called Colombat, preached to the medical profession that, "All women who have reached this critical period of life should withdraw themselves from the vicissitudes of atmospherical influences, lest they

17

promote plethoric accumulations in their regenerative organs which should henceforth be left in a state of inaction''. He was obviously out of touch with women, to say the least, as he is virtually saying that once you're menopausal you should retire from many of life's passions and pleasures. If men had to go through menopause, we'd probably have had a cure for it centuries ago!

Today most experts regard the post-menopausal phase of a woman's life as a potential ''hormone deficiency disease'' which is a far cry from the nihilistic attitudes of doctors such as Colombat.

The evolution of the female species is changing and our average lifespan has increased from a mere 50 years at the turn of this century to 80 years in the 1990s. By the year 2050, it will be 95 years or more and thereafter should continue to increase. Nowadays, the average woman will spend 40% of her life in the post-menopausal state and so you can understand why the long-term problems of the post-menopause have assumed huge medical, social and economic significance.

CHAPTER 4

WHAT CAUSES THE MENOPAUSE?

The word "menopause" means the cessation of menstrual bleeding which is a sign that oestrogen production has fallen to very low levels. It is due to the inability of the ovaries to manufacture the sex hormones, oestrogen and progesterone and can be called ovarian failure.

Why Do The Ovaries Fail?

This is the million dollar question as the human female is the only creature to outlive her sex glands and reproductive capacity. One may well ask, "Why us? Did mother nature go haywire in a cruel twist of fate, or are we simply living longer than God had programmed for us?"

Even though we may wish it didn't happen, the fact is our ovaries simply run out of follicles (eggs) around the age of 50 years. It is follicles within the ovary that produce the vast majority of oestrogen and all the progesterone.

Are Ovaries Of Any Use After The Menopause?

The ovaries after menopause still have an important function because they can still produce very small quantities of oestrogen and significant amounts of testosterone for approximately twelve years[3]. Thus, the ovaries of a menopausal or post-menopausal woman are certainly not dead, dying or useless organs. The issue of whether ovaries should be routinely removed during a hysterectomy in a menopausal woman remains complex and controversial and if you are faced with this decision it is wise to obtain several expert opinions.

After the menopause the adrenal glands continue and indeed may increase their production of hormones that are then converted in your fat (adipose tissue) into oestrogen. This adrenal gland production of oestrogen may continue for up to twenty years after the menopause and varies in amount between individuals, depending upon the amount of fat they have and the health of their adrenal glands. The adrenal glands take over the production of oestrogen from the ovaries after the menopause and heavier women with more adipose tissue have higher total levels of oestrogen than thin women. This is probably the reason why *fat women often appear to age more slowly than very lean women. Thus, there is no benefit in being underweight as we pass through the menopausal years.*

The amount of the male hormone testosterone produced by your ovaries is very significant and continues to be so in the post-menopausal years. The ovary is probably a more potent source of testosterone than the adrenal glands and so contributes greatly to your sexual desire and enjoyment during your post-menopausal years. In women who do not receive oestrogen replacement, the relatively greater amount of testosterone produced by the post-menopausal ovary may lead to an increase in facial hair, thinning of the scalp hair and shrinkage of the breasts.

Do We Have A Simple Test For The Menopause?

The menopausal ovary being devoid of eggs is unable to manufacture significant amounts of the female sex hormones and if a blood test is done at this time to measure the levels of oestrogen and progesterone, they will be found to be at low levels. In menopausal and post-menopausal women blood oestrogen levels, (which are measured in the form of oestradiol) are generally less than 200 pmol/L. The term pmol/L means picomoles per litre and is a standard laboratory measurement, which is a miniscule amount.

The function of the ovaries is under the control of the pituitary gland which is situated at the base of the brain and acts as the master controller for the many hormonal glands in the body. The pituitary gland is very sensitive to the hormonal output of the ovaries and begins to react when the ovaries fail to pump out oestrogen and progesterone into the circulation. The pituitary gland is not at all happy with the failure of the menopausal woman's ovaries and quickly starts to pump out large amounts of a hormonal messenger called **Follicle Stimulating Hormone** (FSH), which travels in the circulation to the flagging ovaries to try and stimulate them back into action. (See diagram 3). Here we can see that mother nature is not perfect and alas the stubborn ovaries have gone on strike forever and despite the hormonal pleas and wooing from the pituitary gland, the ovaries remain dormant. The pituitary gland cannot comprehend that the ovaries are unable to respond to its advances and, in a futile attempt to reawaken them, it continues to pump out ever increasing amounts of FSH into the circulation.

This achieves nothing but does provide a useful diagnostic test for your doctor to assess whether you are menopausal. Typically, blood FSH levels are quite high if you are menopausal with levels being between 40 to 200 mU/L. The term mU/L means milliunits per litre and is a standard laboratory measurement which is a miniscule amount. After the menopause FSH levels increase to 10 to 15 times higher than in pre-menopausal women.

These blood tests can be very useful in women who are suffering with many and vague symptoms for which the doctor can find no obvious cause. Symptoms such as chronic fatigue, rheumatic aches and pains, anxiety,

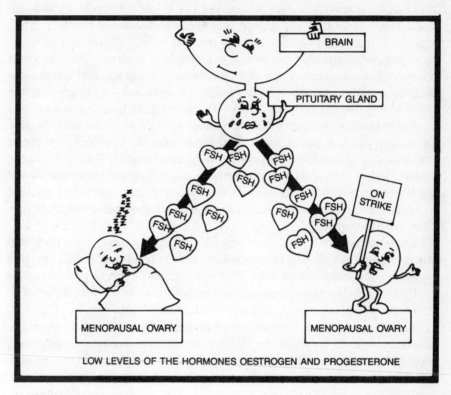

LOW LEVELS OF THE HORMONES OESTROGEN AND PROGESTERONE

DIAGRAM 3

depression and poor libido may be due to a lack of of oestrogen and progesterone which is not uncommon in the years leading up to the menopause. This time of life is called the pre-menopause and though it typically occurs in the late 40s, it may start any time after the age of 35 years. It is often associated with a change in the pattern of the menstrual cycle with menstrual bleeding becoming erratic — less or more frequent or heavier or lighter in amount. During the pre-menopausal years blood tests to measure the levels of oestrogen, progesterone and FSH may be able to pinpoint a lack of oestrogen and progesterone, and, if so, appropriate hormone replacement therapy can be given at this time.

During one of my country trips, a pre-menopausal woman came up to speak with me after I had given a lecture. She had been complaining of hot flushes, anxiety, panic attacks, headaches, neck aches and a total loss of libido.

She had seen several doctors who asked her if her menstruation was still regular and as soon as she replied that she menstruated at monthly intervals the verdict was that she could not possibly be suffering with a deficiency of oestrogen and that her symptoms were due to stress. She was given a prescription for sedatives and anti-inflammatory drugs and told to rest more and cease reading women's magazines. This woman was very angry and was made to feel that she could not cope with the so-called normal phases of life.

A blood test to measure the hormonal levels is a simple and non-invasive procedure and it is also a simple and physiologically appropriate thing to try a course of natural Hormone Replacement Therapy (HRT), for three months at least to see if these pre-menopausal symptoms can be alleviated. Such treatment can be dramatically effective and often avoids the need for sedatives, anti-depressants, painkillers and anti-inflammatory drugs in pre-menopausal women.

Some women are told not to worry about their hormones until they stop menstruating completely, at which time they can return for HRT. By this stage you may have turned into a little wizened up old prune and even your mother can then pronounce you menopausal!; you won't need a doctor to make the diagnosis.

Many body cells need oestrogen to maintain their normal function, for example, the cells of the vagina, bladder, breast, skin, bones, arteries, heart, liver and brain, have oestrogen receptors and require oestrogen to stimulate these receptors for normal cellular function. Loss of the three sex hormones, oestrogen, progesterone and testosterone, may be associated with an increase in heart attacks, high blood pressure, osteoporosis, increased risk of cancer and abnormalities in the brain's chemistry. Hormone replacement therapy has been used for over 40 years to improve the quality and quantity of life for women.

CHAPTER 5

WHAT ARE THE FIRST SYMPTOMS OF MENOPAUSE?

The signs and symptoms that signal a deficiency of oestrogen can be divided into those that occur immediately (acute) and those that occur in the long term (chronic).

EARLY SIGNS

1. Hot Flushes

Probably the most telltale sign of all is the onset of hot flushes, or, as they are called in America, the "hot flashes". You may feel hot and flustered when all around are cool, calm and collected as they complain bitterly when you open windows and turn off heaters. Hot flushes are due to the fact that the body's thermostat situated in the area of the brain known as the hypothalamus does not function at all well without the presence of oestrogen. One minute you may be cold, sweaty and shivering and the next minute you feel like an inferno with an irresistible desire to pull off all your clothes and bedding. One patient told me that her nocturnal hot flushes kept her husband warm all night, so that he no longer needed to turn on the electric blanket.

Nearly 80% of menopausal women are troubled with hot flushes and in 70% of this group the flushes will last, on average, for five years. They vary in severity between different women and may be associated with heart palpitations, dizziness and strange, crawling or itching sensations under the skin.

2. Aches & Pains

Another possible early symptom of oestrogen deficiency is an increase in various bodily aches and pains. For instance, your headaches may become more frequent or severe, your joints may ache, your back and neck may ache and you may begin to suffer with various rheumatic aches and pains.

3. Vaginal Dryness

The vaginal tissues are very sensitive to the effects of oestrogen deficiency and more than 50% of menopausal women are troubled by vaginal dryness and failure to lubricate adequately during sexual intercourse. This causes discomfort or pain during sex and in severe cases may result in some bleeding from the fragile mucous membrane lining the vagina. Without the strengthening effect of oestrogen, the vagina may become more prone to infections with candida and non-specific bacteria which may result in vaginal discharge, itching and burning. In the long term a general shrinkage (atrophy) of the vagina, vaginal opening, vaginal lips (vulva) and clitoris may occur, with a devastating effect upon a woman's sexuality. Hormone Replacement Therapy (HRT) is extremely effective in preventing these changes.

4. Bladder Problems

The tissues of the bladder are also sensitive to oestrogen deficiency and a number of menopausal women complain of the onset of a frequent and/or urgent desire to pass urine, a reduced ability to control the passage of urine (urge or stress incontinence), a reduced bladder capacity and an increased susceptibility to bladder infections (cystitis).

The tissues of the bladder are also sensitive to oestrogen deficiency and a number of menopausal women complain of the onset of a frequent and/or urgent desire to pass urine, a reduced ability to control the passage of urine (urge or stress incontinence), a reduced bladder capacity and an increased susceptibility to bladder infections (cystitis). Oestrogen replacement therapy maintains good pelvic tissues and reduces urinary incontinence.

5. Dry & Ageing Skin

Both the superficial and deeper layers of the skin on our face and body are sensitive to oestrogen as are the collagen fibres criss-crossing in the deeper skin layers. Without oestrogen the skin is more prone to dehydration and irritation and collagen depletion results in the more rapid appearance of wrinkles.

6. Poor Sleep

Oestrogen deficiency can also adversely affect our sleeping patterns so that difficulty going to sleep or early morning waking can set in. Sleeping disorders may be helped by HRT especially if they are associated with hot flushes. Studies have shown that taking oestrogen increases the proportion of sleep spent in the dreaming phase. Many women find that taking oestrogen improves poor memory and decreases irritability which may be in part due to its beneficial effect upon sleep.

WHAT ARE THE FIRST SYMPTOMS OF MENOPAUSE?

The acute symptoms that are characteristic of the oestrogen deficiency of the menopause may be grouped together in a chart and scored according to the following scale:

Absent = 0   Mild = 1   Moderate = 2   Severe = 3

OESTROGEN LEVEL SCORE CHART

OESTROGEN DEFICIENCY SYMPTOMS	SCORE (0-3)
Depression and mood changes	
Anxiety and/or irritability	
Unloved or unwanted feelings	
Poor memory and concentration	
Poor sleeping patterns (insomnia)	
Fatigue	
Backache	
Joint pains, increase in arthritis	
Muscle pains	
New facial hair	
Dry skin and/or sudden wrinkling	
Crawling, itching, burning sensations in the skin	
Reduced sexual desire	
Frequency or burning of urination	
Discomfort during sexual intercourse	
Vaginal dryness	
Hot flushes and/or excessive sweating	
Light-headedness or dizziness	
Headaches	
YOUR TOTAL SCORE:	

TABLE 1

This chart is derived from Professor Nordin's Menopause Questionnaire, Institute of Medical & Veterinary Science, Adelaide, South Australia.

If your total score for all of these symptoms is 15 or more, then it is likely that you are suffering from a deficiency of oestrogen. If your score is around 30, your body is crying out for oestrogen. This can be confirmed or refuted with a simple blood test to check your level of oestrogen and Follicle Stimulating Hormone.

It is an interesting exercise to score your symptoms of oestrogen deficiency before and after commencing Hormone Replacement Therapy. While on HRT your score can be done every 3–4 months and provides a useful self-check of adequate hormone replacement therapy. Do not alter your dosage without first consulting your doctor.

7. Emotional Changes

Mental and emotional changes are common at the time of the menopause, the most common complaints being depression and anxiety. Personality changes may occur with rapidly changing moods, irritability, loss of confidence and panic attacks occurring in women who pre-menopausally had none of these problems. An inability to cope mentally and emotionally is often more poignantly evident in career women with positions of high profile and responsibility. Some women say that they feel numb and can no longer muster any passion or "joie de vivre". If this occurs on a physical level a woman may experience a total loss of libido and in extreme cases she may become sexually frigid.

AND THEN THERE'S . . . YOUR MENTAL ATTITUDE

Your mental attitude is a powerful factor in colouring your personal experience of menopause. Oestrogen deficiency does not affect all women in a negative way and indeed some simply sail through the menopause with no emotional changes. Some women find that the cessation of hormonal highs and lows associated with monthly menstruation makes their menopause a time of tranquillity and composure. Thus, it is dangerous to stereotype menopausal women or we could all be brainwashed into having a midlife crisis!

The common emotional changes associated with the menopause are not always secondary to oestrogen deficiency alone. There may be numerous psycho-social stresses such as adolescent children, caring for elderly parents, coping with the altered self-image of ageing, your husband's midlife crisis and possibly the "empty nest syndrome". All these stresses can exert an emotional, mental and physical toll especially in the caring, giving type of woman who may find that she is continually supporting others, with no one returning her support or praise. If this is your case, I strongly recommend that you indulge in some well deserved self nurturing — e.g. a holiday, a regular massage, tai chi or do something really adventurous!

MALE MIDLIFE CRISIS

We know that men cannot go through a literal menopause. However, for many men the phase of midlife brings significant hormonal changes too, as well as important physical and psychological changes. Put these all together in a melting pot and you may very well have the ingredients for a male midlife crisis. This is undoubtedly one of the reasons why divorce rates soar at this time and many women get the shock of their lives. These women are left in the well known "empty nest syndrome" with hubby fleeing the domestic scene. Conversely, the male not infrequently gets the "nesting syndrome" and spreads his wings with a younger woman finding that her youthfulness rekindles his feelings of manliness and passion and he feels that life is beginning all over again.

This situation is very emotive and can be extremely traumatic. It could probably be averted in many cases if males received more information and supportive counselling especially with their wives, at this time. In some cases, the timely use of testosterone replacement therapy in men, even if only on a temporary basis, can bring back the sparkle into a long-term sexual relationship.

If older men keep running off with younger women what will the women they leave behind do? Well, one obvious strategy is that they can also get the "nesting syndrome" and run off with younger men! I have seen lots of older women do this very thing and have happy relationships. There are statistics to support such behaviour, as menopausal women who take natural oestrogen have been found on average to live nine to ten years longer than their male counterparts. To avoid loneliness in old age a man ten years younger could probably fit the bill very nicely!

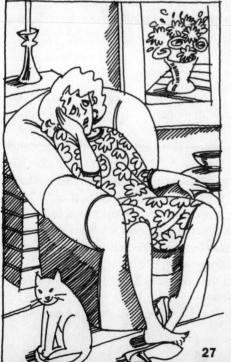

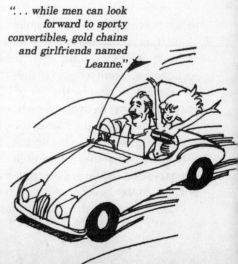

*"We're rapidly approaching the **change of life** when we can look forward to hot flushes, crazy mood swings and chalky bones . . ."*

". . . while men can look forward to sporty convertibles, gold chains and girlfriends named Leanne."

CHAPTER 6

LONG TERM CONSEQUENCES OF OESTROGEN DEFICIENCY

Life expectancy for women today in western civilisation is 80–85 years. The fastest growing segment of such populations is around 85 years and most of these are women. Currently, in the USA there are over 100,000 women over the age of 100.

When a woman becomes menopausal, she can anticipate another 30–40 years of life, so that she passes around 40% of her life span in a post-menopausal state — in other words without sex hormones in her body. Wow! That sounds fairly dramatic, profound and perhaps for the majority of women who love feeling and acting like a woman, a little awesome.

Five years after menopause, most women will have thinning, dryness and shrinkage (atrophy) of the vagina if they don't take oestrogen replacement therapy. For the increasing number of women in their 70s and 80s, who still want to be sexually active, vaginal atrophy is a real concern. However, for such women the biggest problem is not whether to be sexually active, but is finding a partner as most men don't get to 85.

A. Cardiovascular Disease

Forty per cent of Australian and American women will suffer from heart disease or stroke. Up to the time of the menopause, women enjoy a relative protection against cardiovascular disease (diseases of the blood vessels and circulation) compared to their male counterparts and indeed their incidence of heart attacks is only one third that of men. Unfortunately, after the menopause, women begin to lose this relative protection from heart attacks and strokes, so that by the age of 75, they have a similar risk to men. Why do they become prone to disease of their blood vessels after the menopause? This is a very important question in the context that around 45,000 deaths per year occur in the Australian community from heart attacks with a large number of these occurring in post-menopausal women. The most important factor appears to be the loss of oestrogen in the body which results in unfavourable changes in the blood cholesterol levels.

After the menopause the imbalance in cholesterol results in an increase in the process of blockage and hardening of the arteries (atherosclerosis), especially in women who smoke, are obese or sedentary in their lifestyle.

An early menopause is bad news for your cardiovascular system and women who lose the function of their ovaries before the age of 40 have a greater risk of heart disease than women who have a menopause ten years later.

The good news is that large-scale population studies such as the Framingham Study, have proven that giving oestrogen replacement can restore a favourable balance in the cholesterol levels.

The risk of cardiovascular disease can be reduced by approximately 50% in women who are given oestrogen at or soon after the menopause[17]. It is important to note, however, that this only applies if natural oestrogens are used. To put it in a simple way, one could say that if you took two large populations of women and gave one population natural oestrogen for twenty-five to thirty years after the menopause and you didn't give any natural oestrogen to the other population of women, the population that took oestrogen would have half the risk of strokes and heart attacks. This is because oestrogen reduces total cholesterol, increases the good type of cholesterol and prevents cholesterol from being deposited in the walls of the arteries.

We know for sure that oestrogen alone is good for your blood vessels and heart, but we are not sure if adding progesterone to the oestrogen will reduce the benefits of oestrogen upon your cardiovascular system, particularly if such combined HRT is given for many years. We are still searching for the ideal and safe progesterone.

Your risk of future cardiovascular disease is not only determined by the loss of oestrogen. Other risk factors are equally and sometimes more important determinants of cardiovascular disease. These are smoking, high cholesterol, a family history of cardiovascular disease, high blood pressure, a high fat diet and a diet that is deficient in raw foods, fish and liquids, such as water and fresh juices. See Chapter 10 to minimise these risk factors.

THE GOOD NEWS ABOUT LONG TERM USE OF HRT

Now that we are living longer, the possible long-term effects of oestrogen deficiency have become most important. In other words, how may you be affected 25 to 40 years after the menopause if you do not take HRT?

The inaugural scientific meeting of the Australian Menopause Society held in Brisbane in September 1989, came up with some brain-snapping facts. A study of 8,841 women in a Southern Californian retirement community found that women who had used oestrogen replacement therapy had a significantly reduced risk of death from all causes, compared with women who had never received oestrogen. Much of this reduced death rate was due to a marked reduction in the death rate from heart attacks in women on oestrogen. The lowest death rate was seen in the long-term users of oestrogen[4].

At this meeting Professor Henderson from the USA said that taking natural oestrogen led to a 50% to 60% reduction in the risk of heart disease and stroke which gave an extra 4.2 years of life on average.

Another benefit of natural oestrogen cited at the meeting was a lower death rate from same cancers. In particular, HRT appears to reduce the risk of cancer of the ovary by up to 40%.

So, overall in the long term we may be better off taking natural oestrogen than we are without it. Still many women and doctors are reluctant to use adequate doses of oestrogen for sufficient periods of time. The idea of HRT still sparks feelings of danger in Australian women who have one of the lowest rates of HRT usage in the western world. Perhaps this is because they are out of touch and still think about the way HRT used to be twenty years ago when large doses of synthetic oestrogen were given without the proper balance of progesterone. This resulted in a higher incidence of uterine cancer, blood clots and high blood pressure and unfortunately left the wrong impression that all HRT is controversial. This is not so and the natural oestrogens of today are so safe that they cannot be realistically compared to the super-human doses of synthetic oestrogens that were previously given. So please relax. Provided you have all the necessary preliminary tests and examinations, the use of natural oestrogen should only add years to your life as well as greatly improving its quality.

B. Osteoporosis

"If hypertension is a silent killer, osteoporosis is a silent thief. It insidiously robs the skeleton of its banked resources, often for decades, until the bone is weak enough to sustain a spontaneous fracture." F. S. Kaplan, 1983.

Osteoporosis has been called the "silent epidemic" and presently afflicts one in every three women in western civilisation. However, if women take the right precautions early enough this insidious bone-weakening disease is preventable.

Osteoporosis is the abnormal loss of calcium from the bones, which causes them to weaken and become susceptible to fractures (breakage). It was once thought that osteoporosis was simply a normal part of the ageing process and that it should be accepted gracefully because, after all, it was just a manifestation of mother nature. We now know this is not the case. Osteoporosis is a disease that can be avoided in the majority of cases.

Nowadays, no woman should have to suffer its debilitating effects. Epidemiologists predict that by the year 2050 the world will be full of little old ladies, one third of them suffering with osteoporosis. I feel that this is unduly pessimistic as doctors now know how to prevent it. By the year 2050, I believe we will see the good results of preventative medicine reflected in a much lower incidence than the current epidemic.

Currently, osteoporosis is very common; by the age of 60 one in four women living in the western world will have developed a significant degree of bone loss. Most of these women are free of symptoms in the early stages of osteoporosis — so what we're dealing with is indeed a silent epidemic.

By the age of 75, one quarter of all women will have sustained a fracture of the hip. Four in every five fractured hips are associated with osteoporosis. One third of the women who fracture their hips will die within six months.

Fifty per cent of untreated women will have an osteoporotic fracture by 85 years of age.

By now you are probably shaking in your boots, feeling that it would be easier to avoid death and taxes than osteoporosis. Do not despair. By following simple guidelines, osteoporosis can be prevented.

RISK FACTORS FOR OSTEOPOROSIS

There are definite risk factors along the way that tell if you are more likely to develop osteoporosis.

1. Race

The first risk factor is your **race**. If you are fair-skinned or Asian, your chances for osteoporosis are higher than those of Maori, Polynesian and black women, in whom the bones are denser with a slower rate of post-menopausal bone loss.

2. Build

Secondly, your **build** can be a risk factor. Obese women suffer less osteoporosis, so there are some advantages in being overweight. Fat, or adipose tissue, is the main source of the female hormone, oestrogen, after the ovaries have failed in the post-menopausal woman. Being lean and underweight may be glamorous for your image, but is likely to increase your chances for osteoporosis.

3. Smoking

Another major risk factor is **smoking**, which is bad news for your skeleton because it reduces the production of female hormones from the ovaries, thereby increasing calcium and mineral loss from the bones.

4. Medications

Certain **medications** may predispose you to osteoporosis. If you swallow large amounts of antacids containing aluminium over a long time, this may increase the loss of calcium from your bones. It is preferable to take antacids that are free of aluminium — ask your chemist for suitable brands. Cortisone-type drugs, unfortunately rapidly accelerate the loss of calcium from the bones, so you should take cortisone preparations only when absolutely necessary and in the lowest possible dose for the shortest time.

5. Diet — A Vital Role

This was evident to me when I holidayed in Miami Beach in the USA in the early 1970s. Miami Beach was then the retirement haven of middle/upper-class Americans and one would have expected to see a population of happy, relaxed older women enjoying the good life of the American dream. On the contrary, I was shocked to see these older women who seemed to move slowly without vitality and were typified by the dowagers hump on their thoracic spines. They seemed older than their years as they plodded along with the curve of their spines forcing their faces to regard their feet rather than the sunny skies of Miami. Ironically, these women had brought osteoporosis upon themselves while living in the land of plenty because of their long-term consumption of a high amount of animal protein, phosphorus (largely found in processed foods), salt and sugar. A diet like this may increase your risk of osteoporosis because it increases the loss of calcium in the urine and/or disturbs the balance of calcium between the blood and the bones. If you are considering how much animal protein in the diet is safe for your bones, I suggest 3 to 4 servings of red meat, 2 servings of chicken and 4 servings of fish per week.

What I was seeing in the early 70s is now a statistical phenomenon often talked about during conferences on osteoporosis. In western civilisations, osteoporosis is becoming a much bigger problem afflicting ten times as many women as it did in the 50s and appears at a younger age. Experts agree the reasons must be our western lifestyle, diet and increasing life span.

Women who drink a lot of alcohol and caffeine are also increasing their risk of osteoporosis although a modest social intake does not increase the rate of bone mineral loss.

While on the subject of diet, it is relevant to mention that there are two types of osteoporosis. Both types of osteoporosis can be influenced by a poor diet.

Type 1 Osteoporosis: causes a loss of the inner spongy bone (trabecular bone) and is mainly due to a lack of female and male hormones.

Type 2 Osteoporosis: causes a loss of the hard outer bone layer (cortical bone) and is mainly due to imbalances in calcium and Vitamin D.

The amount of oestrogen produced by your body is affected by the amount of calories you consume. Thus, if you are a chronic dieter and consume a very low kilojoule diet, especially if your menstrual periods are infrequent and light, you may suffer with a premature oestrogen deficiency causing a Type 1 osteoporosis.

You will be more likely to suffer with Type 2 osteoporosis if your diet is specifically lacking in calcium and/or Vitamin D. The Australian Recommended Daily Allowances (RDAs) for calcium are set at 800mg for pre-menopausal women and 1,000mg for menopausal and post-menopausal women. It is alarming to find that three-quarters of all women fail to achieve these RDAs. By referring to Page 98 you can help to ensure that you will achieve your RDA of calcium.

The intake of calcium during adolescense and in the twenties is crucial in determining the ultimate (peak) mass that our bones can achieve. Today many adolescent girls are reducing their peak bone mass by stringent dieting and excessive exercise and will increase their risk of osteoporosis in later life. (See Diagram 4).

The ratio of calcium to other minerals in the diet is also important. The balance of calcium to the mineral phosphorus should be 2 to 1. The modern-day western diet contains too much phosphorus so that the balance has tipped in favour of phosphorus 4 to 1. This excess of phosphorus can speed up loss of calcium from the bone. You should aim to reduce the high phosphorus foods in your diet by avoiding those whose labels include ingredients such as phosphoric acid, sodium and potassium phosphate, polyphosphate, pyrophosphate. Generally, phosphorus and its derivatives are found in processed or canned meats, processed cheeses, instant package food, packaged biscuits and pastries, soft fizzy drinks, packaged breads and cereals. At this juncture, you are probably wondering where your nearest Health Food store is located as many of the goods found at your local supermarket or convenience store are loaded with phosphate food additives.

The mineral magnesium is important in helping your body to utilise calcium and if your intake of calcium is raised, your magnesium intake should be raised as well. The ideal calcium to magnesium ratio is 2 to 1, therefore, if you are taking 1,000 mg of calcium you need 500mg of magnesium. It is

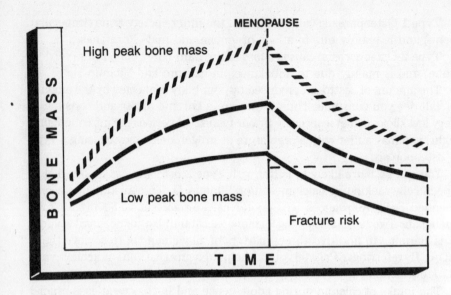

DIAGRAM 4
High peak bone mass provides protection against the consequences of bone loss.

possible to obtain tablets containing both calcium and magnesium in the correct ratio of 2 to 1.

The antioxidant vitamins, Vitamins C and E are necessary for the manufacture and maintenance of the tough fibrous collagen in our bones. Collagen gives our bones flexibility making them less brittle and more resilient to sudden stresses.

A deficiency of Vitamin D may predispose you to osteoporosis and has been found in 30% of post-menopausal women with bone deterioration[1]. Vitamin D is actually a hormone that is synthesised in your skin when it is exposed to direct sunlight, but, many women now avoid the ageing effects of the sun upon their skin. You can obtain Vitamin D from liver, especially fish liver, fatty fish (halibut, mackerel, salmon), butter, eggs and Vitamin D-enriched milk. Women likely to suffer a Vitamin D deficiency are those with food absorption or digestive problems, intolerance to any dietary fat and absence of any exposure to sunlight. In such cases, you should consult your doctor for a blood test to measure your level of Vitamin D and determine your need and dosage of a Vitamin D supplement. Generally speaking, a daily supplement of Vitamin D in a dose of 400 international units is adequate and safe.

6. Exercise

Women who do not carry out regular weight-bearing **exercise** are at far greater risk of developing osteoporosis.

Suitable weight-bearing exercise is not weight-lifting; it is any type of exercise that involves movement in the upright position, so that body weight is being transmitted through the spine, pelvis and legs to the ground, where the force of gravity acts vertically on the skeleton. Ideally, this type of exercise should involve muscular contraction. Suitable weight-bearing exercise is 30 minutes daily of walking, jogging, aerobics or yoga. It is best to choose a form of exercise that you can adopt as a lifestyle. Conversely, too much exercise reduces body fat excessively and particularly if associated with the cessation of regular menstruation, can increase your risk of osteoporosis. Moderation in exercise is the key.

7. Menopause — The Most Important Risk Factor

The loss of production of the female hormones, oestrogen and progesterone, at the time of the menopause is the major cause of osteoporosis.

If women did not go through the menopause, their incidence of osteoporosis would be closer to that found in men (1 in 20). The **earlier the menopause**, the longer a woman spends in the post-menopausal state and the greater her chances of developing osteoporosis. Women who have a premature menopause are at particular risk.

But the women most at risk are those who have had their ovaries surgically removed, especially before they reached the age of 45, and who have never received adequate HRT.

8. Hereditary Factors

Genetic factors are important in determining how dense your bones will become.

Consider yourself at a higher risk than average if your mother, grandmothers or sisters have developed osteoporosis, although you can help to offset this increased risk by ensuring a healthy lifestyle and high calcium diet.

If a woman has several of these risk factors combined, her chances of developing osteoporosis are multiplied. She should do everything possible to remove these risks and decrease her chances. For example, a woman who is thin, has a poor diet, smokes, drinks alcohol excessively, and reaches the menopause before the age of 45 would be a prime candidate for osteoporosis.

OSTEOPOROSIS RISK SCORE
Score your own risk for osteoporosis.

RISK FACTOR	RISK POINTS VALUE	YOUR RISK POINTS

LACK OF MENSTRUATION (AMENORRHOEA) FOR:
      6-12 MONTHS
      12-24 MONTHS
      2- 5 YEARS
      5-10 YEARS
      10 YEARS
(NB. Does not apply if you have had a hysterectomy and are receiving adequate HRT).
	1
	2
	3
	4
	5	

FIRST MENSES AFTER THE AGE OF 17 (LATE PUBERTY)	1	
LONG-TERM USE OF CORTISONE	5	
FAMILY HISTORY OF OSTEOPOROSIS	3	
SMALL FINE-BONED FRAME	2	
CALCIUM DEFICIENCY DURING GROWING PHASE AND/OR LACTATION	2	
TOBACCO USE	1	
IMBALANCE IN EXERCISE, EITHER INACTIVITY OR SUPER-SPORTIVE	2	
RACE: CAUCASIAN OR ASIAN	1	
EXCESSIVE CONSUMPTION OF PROTEIN, SALT, ALCOHOL, CAFFEINE, SOFT DRINKS	1	
OVERACTIVE THYROID, EXCESS THYROXINE	1	
	YOUR TOTAL▶	

TABLE 2

If your score is 9 or more points on this scale, you have a high risk of bone fracture. If your score is 5 to 8 points you have a moderate risk of bone fracture. The most accurate way to determine your risk is to have a bone mineral density test done at the time of the menopause. A bone mineral density test should be a routine screening test for all menopausal women and should be considered as essential as cholesterol measurements, pap smears or mammograms.

THE SIGNS OF OSTEOPOROSIS

Unfortunately in many cases the first sign is often the fracture of a bone, particularly in the wrist, hip or spine, after minimal damage or trauma. To avoid this painful outcome be aware of the signs that may indicate the earlier stages.

1. A gradual reduction in height associated with the lengthening of dresses and slacks.

2. A stooping of the spine and rounding of the shoulders, due to the square-shaped spinal vertebrae gradually collapsing into triangular wedges. If this is allowed to develop some women will form a hump on the spine below the neck, rather disparagingly called a 'dowager's hump'.

3. General aches and pains in the bones may signal early osteoporosis, so remember, all that aches is not necessarily arthritis. Be wary of accepting anti-inflammatory arthritic medication or painkillers without first having tests done for osteoporosis.

4. Another useful clue is the texture of a woman's skin. If it rapidly loses its thickness and suppleness at the time of the menopause, then it is more likely that collagen loss is occurring in the bones. It is the loss of collagen fibres in the dermal layer of the skin that causes sudden wrinkling and loss of texture. Brittle nails and deterioration of the teeth may also give a clue.

According to experts at Kings College, London, the development of osteoporosis is due partly to a loss of collagen in the bones which causes them to become excessively brittle. The loss of collagen in the bones is often mirrored by a loss of collagen in the skin.

IS THERE A RELIABLE TEST FOR OSTEOPOROSIS ?

For the first time, doctors now have a revolutionary test called a "Bone Mineral Density Test" to accurately predict your chances of developing osteoporosis. The Bone Mineral Density Test (BMD) measures the concentration of minerals in your bones to determine how strong and resistant to fracture they are.

Ideally, all women should have a BMD test when they pass through the menopause and not several years later as bone mineral loss can be rapid in the first five years after the menopause. Ask your doctor for a referral to the Department of Nuclear Medicine of your local hospital or a private bone assessment centre to have a BMD test. Ideally, these centres should be equipped with the latest Lunar DPX-L Bone Densitometer machines which utilise dual energy X-ray absorptiometry (DEXA) technology. Measurements of your bone density should be made in the spine and hips. By the way, ordinary X-rays are not an accurate test for osteoporosis.

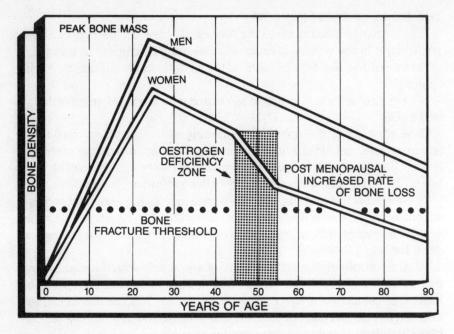

DIAGRAM 5

This test takes only 15 to 20 minutes to perform, does not involve any injections, drugs or discomfort and costs only $50 to $70. It is accurate to within half a per cent and its radiation emission is less than a dentist's X-ray. It really is an ideal test and can put your mind at rest. (See Diagram 5). This diagram illustrates the acceleration of bone loss that occurs when a woman passes into the oestrogen deficiency zone of the menopause. The straight dashed line represents the bone fracture threshold which means that the bone mineral density has become so low that a bone may fracture under the slightest stress. In such unfortunate women, fractures of a hip may occur simply by jumping out of bed and putting all the weight on one hip or a vertebral compression fracture in the spine can occur while sitting in a car travelling over a rough road. Indeed, if your bone density crosses the fracture threshold you become a type of "china doll". From Diagram 5 you can see that the oestrogen deficiency of the time zone around the menopause, represented by the shaded column is a crucial time corridor where loss of bone mass can be greatly accelerated and, indeed, during this time a rapid bone loser can lose a large amount of her total bone mass. *More than 50% of the total amount of bone that will be lost in the post-menopausal years is usually lost in the first seven to ten years after the menopause.* *A new blood test to identify your risk of osteoporosis should become available within the next few years. This is based on the fact that researchers have identified a gene that determines bone strength or density.*

PREVENTION OF OSTEOPOROSIS

The current epidemic of osteoporosis in women aged 60 and above reflects the fact that ten years ago, there wasn't an accurate test to discover the very early stages of this disease. These women came to medical attention only when they had developed humping of the spine or bone fractures and, unfortunately, at this advanced stage, it is difficult to put back the calcium that has been leached out. The good news is that we can prevent calcium from being lost from the bones if treatment is begun in the early stages, at the time of the menopause — and not ten years later.

METHODS OF PREVENTION

1. Hormone Replacement Therapy

HRT is the most effective method of prevention, ideally beginning when deficiency of the female hormones first becomes apparent — usually at the time of the menopause and in some women in the pre-menopausal years. Many studies have shown HRT to be the most effective treatment for the maintenance of bone size and strength and the prevention of bone fractures and HRT is better than any other therapy available for preventing osteoporosis. HRT needs to be given for 15 to 20 years to prevent osteoporosis effectively.

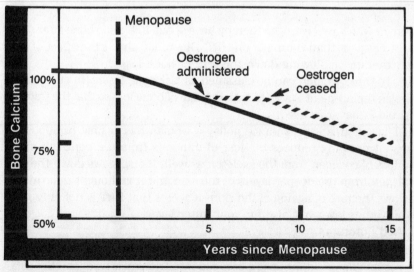

DIAGRAM 6 *Calcium loss following oestrogen deprivation.*

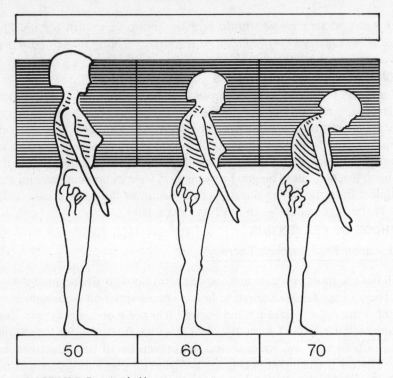

DIAGRAM 7 *Dowager's Hump*

Women who have oestrogen therapy have about 10% more bone after three years' treatment than those not on HRT. Diagram 6 shows the effect of oestrogen therapy in slowing down the rate of bone loss.

One in three women can be classified as fast bone losers. In such cases, oestrogen replacement is able to slow the rate of bone loss so that the fracture threshold is never crossed.

HRT is the greatest insurance policy a woman has against osteoporosis because it not only reduces the loss of minerals from the bone but slows down loss of collagen from the skeleton as well. It also slows down the loss of collagen from the deeper layers of the skin and it is thought that this effect slows the rate of ageing of the skin. It seems that HRT is not only good for your inner layer but also for your outer layer!

HRT And Fractures

The bony vertebrae of the spine may become weak and spongy and their once rectangular solid forms are crushed into triangular wedges. (See Diagram 7). These are called compression fractures. This causes a loss of height, protruding abdomen, curved posture, with compression of the spinal nerves causing sharp shooting pains in the spine and limbs. Currently in Australia, one in four women over the age of 65 years has one or more such spinal compression fractures.

Loss of bone mass also commonly occurs in the hips and there are over 14,000 hip fractures in Australia every year. Without HRT, 50% of post-menopausal women will be at risk of an eventual fracture by the age of 75 years. *Replacement with oestrogen for fifteen years after the menopause extends the age of fracture to 90 years.* Currently, the average life span for Australian and American women is 80 to 85 years and so HRT enables the majority of women to escape fractures. As women continue to live longer, we will need to give HRT for longer periods; the ideal solution would be to re-programme the ovaries to pump out oestrogen indefinitely. Women who use oestrogen therapy have a 60% reduction in the risk of osteoporotic fractures[16].

Some progestagens may have worthwhile ability in reducing bone loss and this provides another reason for combining oestrogens and progestogens in HRT prescriptions.

2. Calcium Supplementation

Calcium plays a role in building up your peak bone mass and reducing bone loss associated with age and menopause. Fracture rates in the elderly are reduced if adequate calcium intake is maintained. Professor Chris Nordin from Adelaide University is a brilliant authority on calcium metabolism and recommends 500mg of calcium daily if you use dairy products regularly, and 1,000mg daily if you do not. Don't forget to use the calcium content of foods on Page 98 to make sure that your diet and calcium supplements provide you with at least 1,000mg of calcium daily. It has been found that less than 40% of menopausal women receive an adequate daily intake of calcium.

Your calcium supplement is best taken *last thing at night* on retiring as it is during sleep and when your stomach is empty that blood calcium levels fall causing parathyroid hormone to dissolve precious calcium from your bones.

I recommend a book called *Allan Borusheks Pocket Calorie Counter*, for those women wanting a useful and excellent guide on cholesterol, calorie and calcium values of foods.

3. Male Hormones (anabolic steroids)

These are well known for their infamous role in competitive sports, yet few know that they are often used to help women with established osteoporosis. The rationale for their use is that menopausal women with high blood levels of testosterone have a slower loss of bone. The role that male hormones play is not clear, but they have been shown to help prevent bone loss and possibly produce some degree of bone gain in established osteoporosis. These injections may be extremely useful for women who are unable to take oestrogen.

Be aware that they may induce an increase in facial hair, greasy skin, pimples, voice deepening and increasing libido so that some women refuse to continue with them. On the other hand, many women find that they reduce musculoskeletal pains, improve skin texture and greatly increase vitality and choose to continue with them.

4. Regular Daily Exercise

Exercising for 30 to 40 minutes every day (see Page 99) is a vitally important strategy to prevent osteoporosis.

EXCITING NEW TREATMENTS

1. Etidronate

This drug is most useful for women with severe osteoporosis or those unable to take oestrogen. It can increase the strength of demineralised bone and reduces the frequency of spinal fractures[2]. Currently, Etidronate is not generally available, but, if you want to know if it can help you, ask your local doctor for a referral to a bone physician or a hospital clinic for bone diseases.

2. Calcitonin

Another natural hormone that may be used more generally in the future is Calcitonin which is extracted from salmon or eels. Calcitonin, used as a nasal spray, delays bone loss both during the menopause and in older women with established osteoporosis. At present, Calcitonin is expensive and needs to be given by daily injection making it unavailable for general use. Hopefully, it will soon be available in the form of a nasal spray and it could become a very useful alternative for the prevention and treatment of osteoporosis, especially for many women unable to take oestrogen replacement therapy.

3. Rocaltrol

This is the active form of natural Vitamin D. A large scientific trial in women with post-menopausal osteoporosis showed that Rocaltrol reduced new spinal fractures by 70% and other fractures by 50% over a three-year period[12]. Rocaltrol is now available on special authority prescription from your doctor if you have established post-menopausal osteoporosis with one or more spinal fractures. If you are started on Rocaltrol, you must not take calcium supplements unless you check with your own doctor first.

All these developments are encouraging but the fact is that modern medicine still does not have the ability to reverse severe established osteoporosis. What doctors can do extremely well is to prevent osteoporosis by the use of treatment in pre-menopausal, menopausal and post-menopausal years. *Do not be lulled into a false sense of security; start taking precautions in your pre-menopausal years and you won't be robbed by the silent thief.*

In Summary

The percentage of older persons in our population is gradually increasing and while today's affluent society has the resources to care for the health of these people, this will not always be so. Epidemiologists estimate that by the year 2025, the percentage of persons under 15 years will have reduced from 35% (in 1901) to 19%, while the percentage of persons over 64 years will have increased from 4% (in 1901) to 16%. (See Table 3).

The smaller number of younger persons will find it increasingly difficult to support financially and socially the health of the larger number of older people. To avoid the high cost for governments and society in providing health care for our ageing population, we must use the tools of preventative medicine while we are in midlife.

Women outlive men and a large number of widows will spend around a decade without their partners. If they cannot maintain mental, emotional and physical health, they may be forced into nursing homes and institutions where health may deteriorate further.

I do not want to sound like a prophet of doom, but rather to help you realise that as a woman you are likely to have a better menopause and post-menopause if you take active responsibility for your mental and physical health.

This means ensuring that your doctor assesses your risk for cardiovascular

CHANGES IN THE PROPORTIONS OF THE YOUNG AND THE ELDERLY IN THE AUSTRALIAN POPULATION FROM 1901 TO 2025

YEAR	POPULATION (IN MILLIONS	PROPORTION <15YR	(%) AGED 64–75YR	>75YR
1901	3.79	35.2	3.0	1.0
1961	10.51	30.2	5.7	2.8
1986	15.97	23.2	6.6	3.9
2005	20.21*	20.9	6.9	5.4
2025	23.86*	19.1	9.5	6.6
*An estimate		Adapted from Economic Planning Advisory Council		

TABLE 3

disease, osteoporosis, cancer and degenerative diseases at the time of your menopause. If such problems are found at this early stage, they can be corrected and further deterioration prevented.

If HRT is given for 10 to 15 years after menopause, we achieve a large reduction in heart attacks, stroke and bone fractures and theoretically such reductions in common diseases of elderly women should become more evident as hormone replacement therapy is continued beyond the age of 65.

Looking at these statistics you may be convinced that every menopausal woman should have HRT. However, this is not necessarily the case as each woman is different. For example, some menopausal women have no worrying symptoms and are not at risk of cardiovascular disease or osteoporosis, as determined by a bone density test and total physical examination. In such low risk women, HRT is not medically necessary. However, you may still decide to take HRT for personal reasons.

Whether or not you and your doctor decide HRT is necessary for you, it will still be wise to begin a lifestyle and nutritional programme of preventative health care for yourself. Strategies like regular exercise, increasing your intake of low fat, high calcium, high fibre foods and raw fruits and vegetables are vital and probably more important than your decision to take hormone replacement therapy alone. For full details on diet, supplements and exercise for midlife and beyond turn to Chapters 10 and 11.

I believe that as women we can become what we visualise ourselves to be. Give yourself positive affirmations that you will be strong, energetic and mentally switched on as you age and work towards these goals every day in a practical way. Don't let anyone else convince you that your health will decline with age as I have witnessed thousands of women improve with age and start to look younger once they began using the miraculous healing tools of naturopathic medicine and a healthy lifestyle.

CHAPTER 7

YOUR VISITS TO THE DOCTOR

Your First Visit

I suggest you consult a doctor or gynaecologist who has a special interest in women's health and a Menopause Clinic or Women's Health Centre is usually your best bet. Your first visit should be around 30 to 40 minutes, thus allowing time for a full history and physical examination.

Your History

Before beginning HRT or deciding that it is not for you, your doctor must take a medical history and perform a full physical checkup and a battery of tests. She will want to know if there are any risk factors in your family history that could influence the decision to begin HRT. For instance, a strong family history of breast cancer occurring in close relatives, especially if diagnosed before the age of the menopause, would cause your doctor to be more conservative in giving you oestrogen replacement. Conversely, a family history of osteoporosis or cardiovascular disease would probably influence her to advise you more strongly to take oestrogen replacement on a long-term basis as this would reduce your chances of following in your female relatives' footsteps. Particular attention should be paid to your menstrual pattern. If you have had irregular bleeding or bleeding after twelve months of stopping regular menstruation then you will need a curettage of the uterus or hysteroscopy before commencing HRT. This will rule out the presence of uterine or cervical cancer which, if discovered, would require urgent treatment.

Your contraceptive needs should also be discussed because, if you are pre-menopausal and wanting to begin HRT before the real onset of the menopause, then theoretically there is still a slight risk of pregnancy. Modern day natural HRT cannot guarantee 100% protection against pregnancy as it is not as effective in suppressing ovulation as the oral contraceptive pill. Thus, in pre-menopausal women or those in the very early stages of menopause while there is still a slight chance of ovulation, the mini pill (progesterone only pill) could be taken every day along with natural oestrogen or a low-dose oral contraceptive pill could be continued until one is certain that menopause has arrived. Alternatively, mechanical methods of contraception such as the diaphragm, intra-uterine contraceptive device or condoms can be used until the menopause has definitely arrived. Generally, doctors recommend that you use some form of contraception until you have had no menstrual periods for a year. After that time you should be able to relax and stop worrying about the fear of pregnancy. It is extremely unlikely you would conceive after over a year without a menstrual period. Also, an elevated FSH level (over 30), see Page 20, would indicate you are menopausal and, therefore, beyond your fertile stage.

A previous history of gynaecological cancer is very significant. If you have had successful treatment of a previous cancer of the ovaries or cervix, then HRT should not be a problem. If you have had successful treatment of a cancer of the inner lining of the uterus (endometrial cancer) taking oestrogen could theoretically stimulate a recurrence. If this applies to you, check with the gynaecologist and cancer specialist (oncologist) who treated your cancer and then make a decision regarding HRT.

Your past history is also worth scrutinising because, if you have had a problem with high blood pressure, heart disease or blood clots, special care will be needed in deciding the type of HRT that is best for you. In such cases the oestrogen patch is likely to be the safest form of HRT. See Page 64.

Your doctor will also want to know about your lifestyle and daily habits as well as your expectations and needs concerning your sex life. Ideally, before starting HRT you should stop smoking, begin to exercise regularly and if overweight, slim down.

Menopausal women who are enjoying an active and fulfilling sex life can optimistically be told that HRT can ensure a lasting quality to this pleasure. It will definitely help vaginal and vulval lubrication, the ability to achieve a satisfying orgasm and prevent shrinkage of the breasts, uterus, vagina and clitoris. Most women want to remain sexually active way beyond the menopause.

Your doctor will also quiz you about your symptoms such as hot flushes, obviously with the intent of assessing your level of oestrogen deficiency. Why not make it easy for him by taking along your completed oestrogen level score chart as on Page 25 of this book.

That Vital Physical Examination

It should take about twenty minutes and will be a complete strip off. Your heart, blood pressure, blood vessels and weight will be checked. The thyroid gland which is that soft fleshy mound in the front of your Adam's apple is pressed along with a thorough feel around in the neck and armpits for lumps and assorted swellings. The breasts should be painstakingly felt for any tenderness, lumpiness or thickenings. The skin and nipples of the breast are also checked. The abdomen is checked, followed by the pelvic examination. The vagina and vulva should be checked for signs of oestrogen deficiency or disease processes. In a woman with oestrogen deficiency the vaginal secretions are scanty and alkaline (non-acidic) and the mucous membrane lining the vulva and vagina may be thin and fragile. Understandably, in such cases the taking of a pap smear may be extremely uncomfortable in which case the use of a vaginal oestrogen cream for one month will be required to restore the vaginal tissues to normal so that a pap smear and pelvic examination can be done comfortably.

You will be asked to cough or bear down while your doctor views the vaginal opening as this reveals any tendency to prolapse of the uterus and bladder. Next comes what I affectionately call the "squeeze test" as the doctor palpates with two hands your uterus, ovaries and surrounding pelvic organs. This is a vital part of your checkup as presently the only early evidence of a cancer of your ovary is a swelling or lump in the pelvis, so try to relax and breathe deeply as it makes the pelvic examination far more accurate. Making sure you have emptied your bladder before your examination is also a great help, especially when your doctor is squeezing around in your pelvis, checking the size and consistency of your uterus.

If your uterus is enlarged or your ovaries are enlarged or difficult to feel because you are overweight or tense, it is wise to have an ultrasound scan of your pelvis. This can reveal uterine fibroids (fibrous growths) or tumours and cysts on the ovaries. Cancer of the ovaries becomes more common during the post-menopausal years and carries a very high risk of death because it produces few symptoms in the early stages. Presently, ovarian cancer is the fifth most common cancer in women and kills twice as many women as cancer of the cervix. It is usually first discovered in women over 45 at a stage when it has spread extensively and can be considered generally as a slow-growing cancer which is not diagnosed until late. An ultrasound scan helps to discover growths on the ovaries in the early and curable stages. The more frequent use of ultrasound scans of the pelvis to check the ovaries in women over 45, will reduce these currently pessimistic statistics.

Special Tests
To help determine your individual requirements for HRT, it is best to have some simple tests. The most important is the breast X-ray or mammogram. If you have an undiagnosed cancer lurking in your breast, taking HRT could

YOUR VISITS TO THE DOCTOR

MENOPAUSE CHECK LIST TABLE

The Physical Examination — Check List

THINGS TO CHECK	LOOKING FOR
HEART, BLOOD PRESSURE, BLOOD VESSELS, VARICOSE VEINS	HIGH OR LOW BLOOD PRESSURE, DISEASES
WEIGHT	UNDER OR OVER
THYROID GLAND	UNDER OR OVERACTIVE, LUMPS
BREASTS	LUMPS, THICKENINGS
ABDOMEN	SWELLINGS, TENDERNESS
PELVIC EXAMINATION	SIZE OF PELVIC ORGANS, CONDITION OF OVARIES, CANCER, PROLAPSE, VAGINAL ATROPHY

Special Tests — Check List

THINGS TO CHECK	LOOKING FOR
PAP SMEAR	PRECANCEROUS OR CANCEROUS CELLS IN THE CERVIX
BREAST X-RAY (MAMMOGRAM)	VERY EARLY SIGNS OF CANCER
BONE MINERAL DENSITY (BMD)	OSTEOPOROSIS
BLOOD TESTS: OESTROGEN, FOLLICLE STIMULATING HORMONE (FSH), BLOOD COUNT, BLOOD SUGAR, LIVER FUNCTION, CHOLESTEROL	YOUR OESTROGEN LEVEL, METABOLIC DISORDERS
URINE TEST	INFECTIONS, KIDNEY DISEASES
PELVIC ULTRASOUND — (IN SELECTED CASES)	DISEASES OF UTERUS AND/OR OVARIES

TABLE 4

theoretically increase its rate of growth. Thus, it is most important to exclude the presence of a breast cancer before beginning HRT and a mammogram is the most accurate means of doing this. Your doctor will examine your breasts very carefully for signs of cancer but even the best doctor in the world can miss a tiny cancer because it is just too small to humanly feel. A good quality low-radiation-dose mammogram can reveal very tiny cancers, as small as one to two millimetres in size long before your doctor can feel them. In Sweden, studies have proven that screening women aged 45 years and over with regular mammograms can reduce the risk of dying from breast cancer by up to 60%.

Routine blood tests to measure your Follicle Stimulating Hormone (FSH), oestrogen level, a full blood count, blood sugar level, liver function tests and blood cholesterol should also be checked. If you have a past history of forming blood clots (thrombosis), then blood should be taken for a clotting factor profile.

Follow-Up Visits

Your doctor will usually make a decision regarding HRT at your second visit during which you can both review and discuss the results of all your tests. The most pressing reason to begin oestrogen replacement without delay would be a poor result on your bone mineral density test, meaning that you are at high risk of osteoporosis. If you feel you need time to think about it or seek a second opinion, you may take several months to sort out your attitude and feelings about HRT. If you decide to start HRT straight away watch its effects by keeping a weekly record of your symptoms on your oestrogen deficiency score chart (see Page 25).

After starting HRT see your doctor after two months, six months and twelve months; thereafter at twelve-monthly intervals. This will enable him to fine-tune your HRT to suit your individual needs. Your general physical examination, pap smear and mammogram should be repeated every twelve months. If your initial bone mineral density test was satisfactory, this can be repeated every three to five years, whereas those women with a low calcium content in their bones should have a bone mineral density test done every one to two years.

If irregular unexplained vaginal bleeding occurs at any time while on HRT, a curettage of the uterus or hysteroscopy should be done by a gynaecologist. Some experts feel that all women on long-term HRT should have more than a pap smear every twelve months. They recommend the addition of a test to take a sample of cells from the lining of the uterus called an endometrial cell sample. This can be done easily at the time of your pap smear and checks for pre-cancerous cells higher up in the uterus above the cervix.

CHAPTER 8

EVERYTHING YOU WILL EVER NEED TO KNOW ABOUT HORMONE REPLACEMENT THERAPY

HRT is an option for every menopausal woman, but the decision to begin should be her own, based on informed choice and individual lifestyle requirements.

WHAT IS THE DIFFERENCE BETWEEN NATURAL AND SYNTHETIC OESTROGEN?

There is a tremendous difference.

Synthetic

Synthetic oestrogens are manufactured in laboratories. They are chemically foreign to the body's metabolic systems and so are not easily broken down by enzymes and can accumulate, causing them to be stronger than the natural oestrogens. For example, the synthetic oestrogen, ethinyloestradiol (brand name Estigyn) is thirty times stronger than the natural oestrogen, oestradiol. The synthetic oestrogens are more likely to cause metabolic changes in the liver leading to an increased incidence of side-effects such as fluid retention, blood clots, aching legs, high blood pressure, etc. I prefer to avoid synthetic oestrogens in menopausal and post-menopausal women as the natural oestrogens are so much safer and are now widely available. Other brands of synthetic oestrogens are Mestranol and Stilboestrol.

Natural

Natural oestrogen is mostly developed in laboratories where an exact chemical replica of your ovaries' oestrogens are cleverly formed. Another popular type of natural oestrogen is called Premarin which is extracted from the urine of pregnant mares. Premarin contains a mixture of natural human-like oestrogens (oestrone sulphate) and some more potent equine (horse) oestrogens. So, one could say Premarin is strictly only natural for horses! In general, Premarin is an excellent form of oestrogen replacement for menopausal women, but, because of its potency it can cause metabolic changes in the liver. It should probably be avoided in women with obesity, high blood pressure, high cholesterol, varicose veins and in smokers.

The most common truly natural oestrogens are:

■ Oestradiol valerate (brand name Progynova, Primogyn Depot).

■ Piperazine oestrone sulphate (brand name Ogen).

■ Oestriol (brand name Ovestin).

■ Micronised oestradiol (brand name Trisequens).

These natural oestrogens are familiar chemicals to our body's metabolic system and are easily broken down into forms that are able to be easily excreted by our livers and kidneys. They do not accumulate in the body and are therefore less likely to cause side effects than the synthetic oestrogens. For these reasons all women on HRT should be using the safer natural oestrogens.

Because natural oestrogens are readily broken down (metabolised) by the body, if they are given in tablet form, they may need to be given twice daily (at 12-hourly intervals) to maintain adequate blood levels of oestrogen during a full 24-hour period. It is not uncommon to see women on a once-a-day tablet of natural oestrogen who complain of hot flushes, dry vagina, fatigue and other symptoms of oestrogen deficiency. Their blood tests often reveal inadequate levels of oestrogen and in such cases they are usually greatly improved by taking their oestrogen tablet at 12-hourly rather than 24-hourly intervals.

THE DIFFERENT WAYS YOU CAN TAKE HRT

Oral Oestrogen and Progesterone (Hormone Tablets)

The most widely used and best known form of HRT is the oral or tablet form and most research into HRT has been done using this form. Most menopausal women are happy to take tablet forms of oestrogen and progesterone on a cyclical basis, much in the same fashion that the oral contraceptive pill is taken. There are many different time and dosage schedules by which hormone tablets can be given. The most important point is that if oestrogen is prescribed to a woman who still has a uterus, progesterone — the other female sex hormone — must also be taken for at least ten to twelve days of every calendar month. This will ensure a regular menstrual bleed and greatly reduce your risk of cancer of the uterus, so that you will have less chance of this cancer than a woman who does not receive HRT. Oestrogen tablets can be taken once or twice daily for twenty-one or twenty-five days with a five-day break between courses, with progesterone tablets being given for the last twelve days of the course. (See Figures A and B).

HORMONE TABLET SCHEDULES

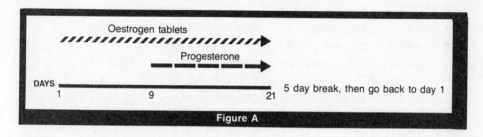

Figure A

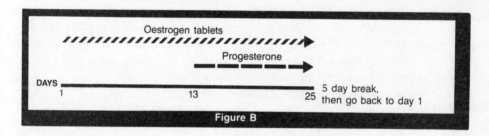

Figure B

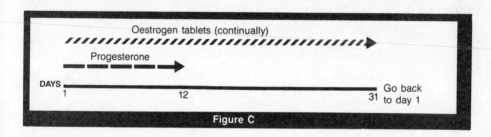

Figure C

Your menstrual bleeding will usually occur during the five-day break from the oestrogen tablets. Some women feel better having a five-day break from oestrogen but if you don't, then there is no harm in taking oestrogen every day. In fact, taking oestrogen every day is safer for your bones and blood vessels and is free of risk provided you add in your progesterone tablets for at least 12 days of each calendar month (See Figure C).

CAN MENSTRUAL BLEEDING BE AVOIDED?

My catch phrase for the 1990s is "designer HRT". This refers to the fact that today every woman who wants HRT can have it tailor made or designed to suit her unique needs. A lot of older post-menopausal women stop HRT because they don't want monthly menstrual bleeding. This is a pity as designer HRT can reduce or completely eliminate menstrual bleeding.

Nowadays older women are often prescribed **both** an oestrogen and progesterone tablet every day without a break which completely avoids menstrual bleeding. We'll soon have a single HRT pill combining the two sex hormones oestrogen and progesterone which can be taken every day without a break avoiding any menstrual bleeding. If any spotting or breakthrough bleeding occurs on this programme you may take a seven-day break from the oestrogen and progesterone tablets every three months which would enable your uterus to shed any built-up lining in the form of a light menstrual period. Some women feel more comfortable having a menstrual bleed every three or so months, seeing it as a "spring clean" for the uterus after which they often feel better. We now have a combined HRT pill called Trisequens containing both oestrogen and progesterone which some women find more convenient and economical than taking two separate tablets.

In women over the age of 65, if it is thought necessary to begin HRT for the first time to slow the progression of osteoporosis, a small dose of oestrogen may be given continuously with no breaks at all. In such cases, a light menstrual bleed can be brought on only two or three times a year by taking a two-week course of progesterone tablets. This reduces the annoyance of

BRAND NAME	CHEMICAL NAME	TYPE	DAILY dose range (mg)	DAILY Minimum Dose to Prevent Osteoporosis (mg)
ESTIGYN	ETHINYL-OESTRADIOL	SYNTHETIC	0.01–0.03	0.02
PREMARIN	CONJUGATED EQUINE OESTROGEN	SEMI-NATURAL	0.3–1.25	0.625
PROGYNOVA	OESTRADIOL VALERATE	NATURAL	1–4	2.0
OGEN	PIPERAZINE OESTRONE SULPHATE	NATURAL	0.625–2.5	1.25
OVESTIN	OESTRIOL	NATURAL	1–4	2
TRISEQUENS	MICRONISED OESTRADIOL	NATURAL	1–4	2

TABLE 5

regular monthly bleeds in older women. A small dose oestrogen patch is a very safe and gentle way of giving HRT to older women (see Page 64).

From Table 5 you can see that daily dosages of oestrogen tablets vary considerably in amount, depending upon how rapidly your enzymes break them down and also upon which brand of oestrogen you are prescribed. For example, Ogen is three times stronger than Ovestin, Progynova is ten times stronger than Ovestin and Estigyn is three hundred times stronger than Ovestin. In all cases you must be guided by your own doctor in finding your required dose. Perimenopausal women still produce their own hormones erratically and generally need higher doses of HRT than older women in their late 50s or 60s.

EVERY WOMAN IS DIFFERENT

One woman's needs may be two to four times higher than anothers. Curiously enough, it is often the woman with a thin, lean build who needs greater amounts of oestrogen because she has very little production of oestrogen from her fatty tissues. Furthermore, it is the lean fine-boned woman who has a greater risk of osteoporosis and will need an adequate amount of oestrogen to prevent this. (See Table 5).

Modern-day HRT has become so safe and effective in the prevention of many problems that every menopausal woman should be considered a candidate for it. If no medical risks exist, HRT should be offered as an informed option. Notwithstanding this, it is still true that menopausal women differ in their need for HRT. Some cannot live without it saying that they feel ancient, decrepit and lifeless without it, while others hardly seem to notice when their ovaries finally stop producing oestrogen.

A minority of menopausal and post-menopausal women actually feel worse on HRT even after all different forms and dosages have been tried. Such was the story of Mandy, a 55-year-old big boned somewhat obese woman who complained of gaining 8kg in weight, fluid retention, aching legs and fatigue since beginning HRT three years ago. Her blood pressure was raised and her legs were bulging with varicose veins. Mandy had been started on hormone tablets at the time of her natural menopause without any blood tests or bone mineral density check being done to assess her individual need and dosage of oestrogen. I checked her bone mineral density and found it to be excellent at over 100%, she had no risk factors for osteoporosis; in particular, her mother had lived to 98 years of age with no trace of osteoporosis or cardiovascular disease.

Thus, it was not essential for Mandy to take HRT and indeed in her case, its side-effects were greater than its benefit. She stopped HRT and six months later had lost 6kg in weight and regained her normal blood pressure and generally felt much better. All Mandy needed was a doctor's permission to stop HRT under the assurance that her bones and blood vessels would be regularly checked to make sure that she would not increase her risk of osteoporosis and cardiovascular disease by not taking oestrogen. In my opinion, Mandy would probably do better without HRT.

Menopausal women should not be made to feel they must take HRT or terrible things will happen, but rather given an informed option as the merits of HRT vary between individuals.

PROGESTERONE — THE BALANCING HORMONE

The ovary makes two different female sex hormones, oestrogen and progesterone. Progesterone balances the effects of oestrogen upon the uterus and is necessary to produce regular periods.

In women with a uterus, if oestrogen replacement is given it is universally accepted that a progesterone must be given for at least ten to twelve days every calendar month to prevent uterine cancer. If oestrogen is taken alone there is an increased risk of cancer of the uterus. It is most reassuring to know that if progesterone is added to oestrogen in women with a uterus, the risk of uterine cancer decreases to less than that in women not on HRT!

Opinion among the experts is somewhat divided as to the necessity of adding some progesterone to oestrogen replacement in women **without a uterus** (hysterectomised women). Some studies show that progesterone given for twelve or more days each month may exert a protective role against breast cancer, but this debate continues and the protective role of progesterone is not proven. I personally do not recommend progesterone tablets to women without a uterus.

Unfortunately, natural progesterone is not effective if taken in tablet (oral) form as it is destroyed by the liver. Currently, the progesterone tablets that are used along with oestrogen in HRT are synthetic progesterone. Synthetic forms of progesterone are called progestagens. Progestagens are not as good as natural progesterone because they don't quite fit the progesterone receptors on your cells. They do however balance the effect of oestrogen upon the uterus, thereby protecting you from uterine cancer.

Some of the progestagens currently used can have unfavourable effects on your cholesterol (see Table 6) and this could reduce the good effect of oestrogen upon your blood vessels. While the debate continues, it is best to be guided by your own doctor and use a progestagen such as Provera or Duphaston that will not cause ill-effects upon your cholesterol balance.

Some women refuse to take any progestagen tablets because they get

TABLE OF PROGESTERONE

BRAND NAME	CHEMICAL NAME	TYPE	DAILY dose range (mg)	ADVANTAGES	DISADVANTAGES
PROVERA TABLETS	MEDROXY-PROGESTERONE ACETATE	SYNTHETIC	2.5–10	DOES NOT CAUSE ADVERSE EFFECTS ON CHOLESTEROL.	MAY CAUSE PMS TYPE SYMPTOMS IN EXCESSIVE DOSAGE.
PRIMOLUT N MICRONOR NORIDAY TABLETS	NORETHISTERONE	SYNTHETIC	0.35–5	MAY REDUCE BREAST TENDERNESS.	MAY EXERT MASCULINE EFFECTS, BUT GENERALLY LESS THAN LEVONORGESTREL. MAY CAUSE ADVERSE EFFECT ON CHOLESTEROL.
MICROVAL MICROLUT TABLETS	LEVONORGESTREL	SYNTHETIC	0.03–0.09		MAY CAUSE ADVERSE EFFECT ON CHOLESTEROL. MAY EXERT MASCULINE EFFECTS.
MICRONISED PROGESTERONE TABLETS	NOT AVAILABLE IN AUSTRALIA	NATURAL	200–300	NO RECOGNISED SIDE EFFECTS. NO ILL EFFECTS ON CHOLESTEROL.	EXPENSIVE. ABSORPTION MAY BE POOR.
DUPHASTON TABLETS	DYDROGESTRONE	SEMI-NATURAL (NEUTRAL)	10–20	GENERALLY LESS SIDE EFFECTS. DOES NOT CAUSE ADVERSE EFFECTS ON CHOLESTEROL.	EXPENSIVE, UNLESS YOU HAVE ENDOMETRIOSIS.
PROGESTERONE PATCHES	NOT AVAILABLE IN MOST COUNTRIES	NATURAL OR SYNTHETIC	NOT DETER-MINED	LESS SIDE EFFECTS. MOST NATURAL WAY OF GIVING PROGESTERONE.	NOT GENERALLY AVAILABLE. EXPENSIVE. SKIN SENSITIVITY.
ANDROCUR TABLETS	CYPROTERONE ACETATE	SYNTHETIC	1–10	REDUCES FACIAL HAIR AND ACNE. IMPROVES SKIN TEXTURE.	IF DOSE TOO HIGH MAY CAUSE FATIGUE, DEPRESSION AND LOSS OF LIBIDO.
PROLUTON DEPOT INJECTION	HYDROXY PROGESTERONE HEXANOATE	SEMI-NATURAL (NEUTRAL)	NOT APPL-ICABLE. GIVE ONE INJECTION EVERY 4–6 WEEKS INTO BUTTOCKS	GENERALLY NO SIDE EFFECTS.	INJECTION SITE MAY BE TENDER FOR SEVERAL DAYS.

TABLE 6

FOOTNOTE **PROGESTAGEN** = SYNTHETIC PROGESTERONE   **PROGESTERONE** = NATURAL PROGESTERONE annoying side effects such as irritability, depression, headaches, weight gain, pelvic pain and bloating. If such side effects are intolerable, progestagen tablets can be safely left off in hysterectomised women or progesterone injections (Proluton Depot injections) can be given every four to six weeks. In my experience, these progesterone injections are very well tolerated and generally free of side effects. Proluton Depot injection acts in a similar way to progestagen tablets in regulating the menstrual cycle and brings on a regular menstrual bleed.

Patches containing either synthetic or natural progesterone may soon be available, and these may be a good alternative for women unhappy with progestagen tablets. If you find that you are unable to tolerate the side effects that progestagens may produce you can ask your doctor's permission to leave them off completely, but you will need to have your uterine lining (endometrium) checked every twelve months with a hysteroscopy. As a last resort you could consider a hysterectomy, but this is not without risk.

HORMONE REPLACEMENT THERAPY IN MENOPAUSAL WOMEN WITHOUT A UTERUS

Approximately 1 in 3 Australian and American women will have a hysterectomy by the age of 65 years. The menopausal woman who has had a hysterectomy is the easiest to treat. In such cases, experts agree that progestagen tablets are not necessary, unless there is a past history of endometriosis which could be reactivated by oestrogen replacement therapy if insufficient progesterone is not given to balance the oestrogen therapy. In women with a past history of endometriosis (whether they have a uterus or not) a low dose continual progesterone tablet should be given along with oestrogen replacement therapy.

If there is no past history of endometriosis, oestrogen therapy can be given by itself in the form of oestrogen tablets, patches, injections or implants.

Some women find that after hysterectomy, their ovaries do not work as well and they may complain of symptoms typical of oestrogen deficiency — in other words, the hysterectomy has reduced the blood supply to the remaining ovaries and thus the ovaries no longer pump out adequate amounts of sex hormones. Such women can be called pre-menopausal.

If this is your case, do the score chart on Page 25 of this book and if your score is around 20, ask your doctor for a blood test to measure levels of FSH, oestrogen and testosterone. If your FSH levels are raised and your oestrogen and testosterone levels are low, then your body is low in sex hormones. This may produce fatigue, depression, aches and pains and loss of libido. A significant number of women in this situation find that hormone tablets do not alleviate these symptoms and will need to take either oestrogen or oestrogen and testosterone in a non-tablet form, such as patches, injections or implants. If these types of HRT are considered, then you may find that your mental, physical and sexual wellbeing soars to new heights, often much better than before your hysterectomy.

If you have had an endometrial ablation, you may still have some remnants of the uterine lining (endometrium) left behind and will need progesterone tablets to balance the effects of your oestrogen replacement therapy upon the endometrium.

Hormone Injections

HRT is also available in the form of injections and these were first manufactured and used in the 1930s and 1940s by German scientists and doctors. The injectable forms of hormones have proven to be popular among European women since the 1950s. They have been used to a small degree only by doctors in America and Australia. Doctors in Australia have probably been unaware of these injectable forms of HRT because they are not promoted at all by drug companies and clinical research material on their use is not widely available. Furthermore, some doctors feel that absorption from these injections is erratic with large fluctuations in the levels of hormones in the blood being produced. Nevertheless, they continue to be popular in Europe.

I feel that there is a role for injectable forms of natural hormones and although I do not think they are the first choice for all women, I have found that for some they can be more suitable than tablet forms.

I myself am a migraine sufferer and cannot take tablet forms of oestrogen. Indeed, oestrogen tablets both of the synthetic and natural form greatly aggravated my migraines producing the classical visual auras of flashing lights and blurred vision. After a hysterectomy for fibroids, I found that my ovaries became pre-menopausal and did not produce sufficient amounts of oestrogen. I began receiving fortnightly injections of natural oestrogen into my buttocks and found that for me they really ''did the trick''. They relieved my fatigue, loss of enthusiasm, aches and pains and frequent headaches. My shrinking breasts became fuller, my libido returned and my acne disappeared. I found that they produced a steady release of that wonderful hormone oestrogen into my blood provided I received them on a regular fortnightly basis. To my relief, they were not painful. (Doctors are generally the biggest cowards and worst patients of all!) I did find that the injection technique is most important and that the needle should be placed deeply into the upper outer part (which is the area with the most fat) of the buttocks. With this technique, the injection produced a slight dull stinging sensation lasting five to ten minutes, which was a small price to pay for the wonderful mental and physical wellbeing that was provided. The natural female hormones oestrogen and progesterone and the male hormone testosterone are available in injection form and are summarised for you in Table 7.

I first learnt of oestrogen injections when a remarkable New York journalist popped into my surgery one day to get her 'fix', as she called it, of Primogyn Depot. Melanie was a woman in her early sixties and looked at

NATURAL HORMONE INJECTION TABLE

TYPE OF HORMONE	BRAND NAME OF INJECTION	FREQUENCY OF INJECTION	USES
Oestrogen (oestradiol valerate)	Primogyn Depot	One injection every two weeks	1. Menopause and Pre-menopause Premature menopause 2. Oestrogen deficiency after hysterectomy 3. Oestrogen deficiency after surgical removal of the ovaries 4. Some severe cases of premenstrual syndrome (PMS) and postnatal depression
Progesterone (hydroxy progestrone hexanoate)	Proluton Depot	One injection every four weeks at mid-cycle	1. Menopause in women unable to tolerate oral progestragens 2. Premenstrual syndrome 3. Postnatal depression
Oestrogen and Testosterone combination	Primodian Depot	One injection every four to six weeks. Some women only require one injection two to three times per year	1. Best used on a temporary or intermittent basis to treat difficult menopausal symptoms, hormonal deficiency after hysterectomy or removal of the ovaries 2. Loss of libido, frigidity and poor marital relationships 3. Severe postnatal depression NOTE: Testosterone is a male hormone and if excessive doses are used, masculine changes may occur, e.g. facial hair and deepening of the voice

TABLE 7
FOOTNOTE: Progesterone must always be given with oestrogen in women who still have a uterus.

Depot = storage injection which is long acting, lasting approximately 3 to 4 weeks in its effects.

least twenty years younger as she related in her vivacious, extroverted way that she had been having one injection every month since her hysterectomy thirty years ago. She was in excellent health and her bone mineral density test did not reveal any signs of osteoporosis. This episode increased my interest in the usefulness of hormone injections for which I am eternally grateful to Melanie; because they were not discussed at all during the medical curriculum at university or teaching hospitals.

Any doctor concerned with the wellbeing of menopausal women will realise that every woman is an individual and that it may be necessary to try different forms and dosages of HRT before physical and mental wellbeing can be restored.

HOW HORMONE INJECTIONS TRANSFORMED TWO WOMEN'S LIVES

Miranda, aged 51 years, came to see me in a very distressed state. She had been on a standard dose of hormone tablets for two years but still complained of a dry itchy vagina, poor libido, headaches, mood changes, insomnia, loss of confidence and black depression. She was very frightened by these uncharacteristic changes in herself and felt she was becoming dependent upon sedatives. Her male psychiatrist told her that it was not her hormones playing up as she was on oestrogen tablets and that she should give up working and concentrate more on her husband's needs. He prescribed a large dose of anti-depressant drugs and told her she would need them to lead a normal life.

Miranda had scratched her vagina and vulva to the point of it developing dry cracks (fissures) and it would often bleed after attempted intercourse. Her blood tests revealed lowish levels of oestrogen so I asked her to double her dose of oestrogen tablets and use a vaginal oestrogen cream. After three months on this increased dosage she returned complaining of a worsening of her migraines and slight improvement only in her itchy, dry vagina. Her fits of deep depression persisted and her marital situation had deteriorated. I then suggested that her liver was probably very active in breaking down the oestrogen tablets and that only small amounts of oestrogen were getting past the liver to the rest of her body which was still crying out for oestrogen. We decided to try a course of natural oestrogen and testosterone injections called Primodian Depot (See Table 7). This was injected every four weeks and a course of progesterone tablets for ten days every month was also given to ensure that a regular menstrual bleed occurred. One month after the first Primodian injection Miranda returned asking for another injection. She was delighted with the first injection that had given her a 90% improvement in all her symptoms. Her vagina had become moist and responsive, her libido was fantastic, her depression had lifted and her husband had been relieved to rediscover the girl he had married. She had felt like socialising again, rejoining her exercise classes and her mental efficiency at work had improved in leaps and bounds. Miranda received a course of three Primodian injections and then we decided to insert an implant of natural oestrogen and testosterone into the fat of her buttocks. She requires an implant every nine to twelve months and has never looked back. Her marriage has been saved, she has thrown out her sedatives and anti-depressants and continues to enjoy her high-powered job. Yes, this is one of many success stories demonstrating that time, patience and confidence in using the correct type of HRT for each **individual** woman will usually work.

Miranda was one of the significant percentage of women who do not find relief from oestrogen deficiency symptoms with oestrogen tablets. These women should not be patronised and told they have a mental or emotional problem or made to feel inadequate. Rather, they should be offered alternative forms of HRT such as injections, implants or patches of oestrogen. If their doctor is not confident in this area, appropriate referral to a Women's Health Centre or Menopause Clinic should be given.

Another interesting story is that of 43-year-old Selina who came to see me because of increasing pre-menstrual syndrome and a total loss of interest in sex. Selina craved more emotional and romantic attention from her 58-year-old husband who was unable to give her this because he resented her inability to fulfill his sexual appetite. They had been married when Selina was 32 and things had been perfect until she had her tubes clipped (a surgical sterilization) at the age of 35 after the birth of her second child. From that point on, Selina began to experience symptoms of gradually increasing oestrogen and testosterone deficiency noting sudden mood changes, loss of sexuality and a reduction in the amount and frequency of her menstrual bleeding. A sample of Selina's blood revealed low pre-menopausal oestrogen and very low testosterone levels. To worsen matters, the amount of sex hormone binding globulin (SHBG) she produced from her liver was very high. Sex-hormone binding globulin is a protein in the blood that carries and binds the sex hormones, oestrogen, progesterone and testosterone. Sex hormones are inactive when they are bound to sex hormone binding globulin (SHBG) and so large amounts of SHBG reduces the active role that sex hormones can play in your body. So this was Selina's dilemma, low amounts of sex hormones and a high amount of sex hormone binding globulin circulating around in her body; she did not stand a chance and things would only get worse as she got closer to the menopause.

Selina and I designed a six-month programme of oestrogen and progesterone tablets but she returned after four months saying that her pre-menstrual irritability and sexual disinterest persisted. We then began a six-month course of monthly natural hormone depot injections. Selina received an injection of Primodian Depot (oestrogen and testosterone) at the end of every menstrual bleed and one Primogyn (oestrogen) and one Proluton Depot (progesterone) injection on day 16 of every menstrual cycle. This produced a dramatic improvement in her mental, physical and sexual wellbeing and her husband could hardly keep up with this new energetic and sexual woman. The combination of these three types of injections containing natural oestrogen, testosterone and progesterone had provided Selina's brain, genital organs and other sexually responsive body cells with sex hormones that her own pre-menopausal ovaries could not provide. After six months Selina found a slight increase in facial hair so we stopped the Primodian injections which contain testosterone. She eventually opted for an implant of natural oestrogen without any testosterone as her libido had returned to normal and she did not want any increase in facial hair. Selina's case illustrates one of the many flexible programmes of "designer HRT" that can be tried for women with hormonal imbalances in the pre-menopausal years.

The injectable forms of natural hormones are very useful for what I call a "hormonal crisis". A hormone crisis is a severe and/or sudden deficiency in hormones that may sometimes occur after a hysterectomy, surgical removal of the ovaries, tubal ligation (surgical sterilization), sudden onset of the menopause, premature menopause, severe medical illness, severe stress, chemotherapy for cancer or after childbirth. Natural hormone injections can truly work wonders and can prevent a hormone crisis leading you into a deep, dark pit; indeed they usually take you quickly and smartly out of the pit. You may only need them for three to six months after which time your own hormones may recover or you will probably find it more convenient to have either an oestrogen implant, oestrogen patch or the more conventional tablet forms of HRT.

Oestrogen Patches

Who ever would have thought that one day we would come up with the idea of applying sticky band aids containing oestrogen to our skin to help us remain well and feminine. The idea is here to stay and Swiss women, American women and the British have been using the patch for nearly a decade. Because of red tape and bureaucratic bungling, Australia has lagged behind as far as the oestrogen patch is concerned, however it has arrived, and is available from your doctor.

The natural oestrogen in the patch is absorbed through the skin into the blood stream and one patch can be worn for three days. The site selected should be one at which little wrinkling of the skin occurs during movement of the body e.g., the lower abdomen, buttocks or lower back. There is no need to have a break from using the patches and in women with a uterus, progesterone tablets should be given for ten to twelve days every month. Hopefully, in the near future we will have patches containing natural progesterone which will be used along with the natural oestrogen patch.

Estraderm patches are available in 3 sizes.

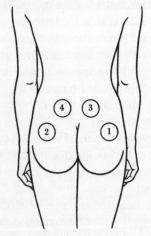

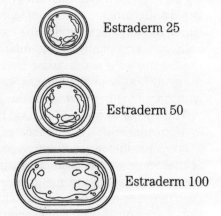

Estraderm 25

Estraderm 50

Estraderm 100

Suggested application sites
of Estraderm patches:
   1 & 2 first week
   3 & 4 second week
   1 & 2 third week etc

Oestrogen patches come in three strengths (25, 50 and 100) and contain the natural oestrogen, oestradiol. Occasionally, the patches can produce skin irritation and redness and this can be reduced by changing the site of the patch with each successive application. Also you may use a Vitamin E or cortisone cream on the skin irritation after removing the patch. In a small number of women the patch produces severe skin irritation and allergy which necessitates changing to another form of HRT.

When the oestrogen patch first appeared on the scene, there was some scepticism about its ability to produce adequate blood levels of oestradiol. However, the patches have undergone extensive testing and have been shown to produce very adequate blood levels of oestradiol, indeed similar to those found in younger pre-menopausal women who still have natural menstrual cycles. A recent study reported in Britain's *Lancet* Medical Journal produced very exciting news about the ability of the oestrogen patch to reduce calcium loss from the spinal vertebrae and hips. The 50mcg oestrogen patch was found to be just as effective as tablet forms of oestrogen in the prevention of osteoporosis[7]. The oestrogen patch is a very safe way for you to achieve constant and normal levels of oestrogen in your blood. Because the oestrogen is absorbed directly into the blood stream it is able to reach your cells before it is broken down by the liver enzymes. Thus, smaller doses of oestrogen can be used in the patch and are far less likely to produce side effects due to metabolic changes in the liver. This makes the patches excellent for women with high blood pressure, fluid retention, bloating, varicose veins, obesity and a past history of clots or thrombosis.

Take the case of Alice, a 62-year-old woman who had been told that she could never take oestrogen because she had suffered two serious blood clots in her leg after her hysterectomy at the age of 43 and again after an appendicectomy at the age of 49. Alice was following in her mother's footsteps as far as osteoporosis was concerned and by the age of 58 had developed an obvious hump on her back. X-rays revealed several crushed vertebrae in her thoracic spine and her bone density values were very low and getting worse every year. Alice knew she needed oestrogen but was too scared to take it for fear that it may cause a recurrence of her blood clots. I prescribed the oestrogen patch for Alice and she began using it regularly. She was greatly relieved to be able to take a form of oestrogen that was safe and effective and we both relaxed when her tests showed six months later that she had stopped losing calcium from her spine.

The oestrogen patch is a godsend to women unable to tolerate tablets or implants of oestrogen. It is also better for high risk women such as those with liver disorders, high blood pressure, varicose veins, thrombosis and those who cannot stop smoking. The patch is also useful for women with bowel problems (e.g. Crohns disease, ulcerative colitis, irritable bowel syndrome and poor intestinal absorption) as in such cases hormone tablets may be poorly absorbed.

Vaginal Oestrogen

Oestrogen can be given via your vagina and indeed this is a very popular form of HRT. It is particularly useful if you have a lot of vaginal dryness or shrinkage and will also reduce bladder problems such as frequency, incontinence or burning. Oestrogen cream is easily inserted with a vaginal applicator which enables you to place the cream high into the vagina (see Diagram 8a). It is best done last thing at night on retiring, after sex, and after emptying your bladder. Oestrogen will be rapidly absorbed through the vaginal lining into the bloodstream and reasonable levels of blood oestrogens can be achieved. Generally, vaginal oestrogen cream is prescribed for once a week usage, but you may use it more often if you desire. If you still have your uterus, frequent and regular use of vaginal oestrogen should be accompanied by a twelve-day course of progesterone tablets every two or three months to guard against oestrogenic over-stimulation of the uterus. These progesterone tablets may bring on a light menstrual period.

Some women find the vaginal oestrogens are satisfactory and do not take any other forms of oestrogen, and several women have told me that they feel very sexy several hours after using these creams! Others find the vaginal creams a little messy and prefer to use vaginal oestrogen pessaries which are inserted high into the vagina with an applicator. Oestrogen tablets can be inserted into the vagina and if placed high in the vagina, are well absorbed. One brand called Vagifem tablets comes with an easy to use vaginal applicator.

If you find that oestrogen tablets taken orally are causing side effects such as nausea or fluid retention, you may find that by changing to the vaginal route of administration for your tablet, you no longer have these side effects. Oestrogen will soon also be available in the form of a ring-shaped pessary that enables oestrogen to be absorbed from the vagina for a longer period. The ring sits high up in the vagina in much the same way as a vaginal diaphragm and its contained oestrogen is gradually absorbed from the ring.

Hormone Implants

Implants of the natural oestrogen, oestradiol have been used for over forty years, but their use has only recently become popular in Australia and is not very common in the USA. The implants consist of small pellets of pure crystalline oestradiol and resemble a tiny piece of spaghetti. They come in various strengths to suit individual needs and are somewhat expensive, although the cost can be claimed from some private health funds. They can be painlessly implanted into the fatty layer of your abdomen or buttocks under a local anaesthetic and many doctors use a small hollow tube with a sharp

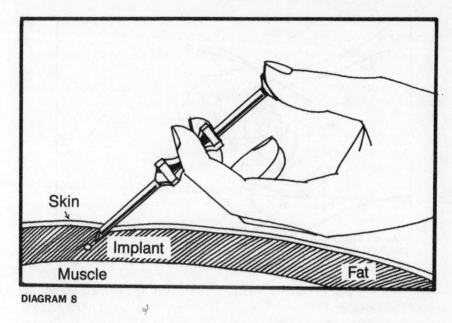

Skin

Implant

Muscle   Fat

DIAGRAM 8

cutting edge to slide the pellet neatly into your fat. (See Diagram 8)

Depending upon the strength of the implant chosen by your doctor, an implant will continue to release oestrogen directly into your blood stream for between four to twelve months which is great for those who cannot remember to take tablets.

Of all the types of HRT, an implant comes closest to copying the function of your own ovaries as in both cases oestrogen is released directly into the bloodstream and carried to the various oestrogen-dependent tissues of your body. Thus, your hungry cells get their supply of precious oestrogen before the liver enzymes can break it down. Unfortunately, this is not so with oestrogen tablets which are first broken down during passage through the liver after their absorption from the gut. Thus, the liver could be said to weaken the effect of oestrogen tablets upon your cells, whereas the oestrogen implant is able to deliver an unweakened supply of oestrogen.

Janet, a 56-year-old woman was having a stressful menopause despite taking oestrogen and progesterone tablets regularly. Her hot flushes and sweats made her feel dirty, her clothes clung to her flesh and she felt as if ants were crawling under her skin. Her libido had vanished and a deep depression had set in. Janet was told that these symptoms were all in her mind and that she needed a good psychiatrist. A blood test revealed low levels of oestradiol and testosterone and we decided to give her an oestrogen and

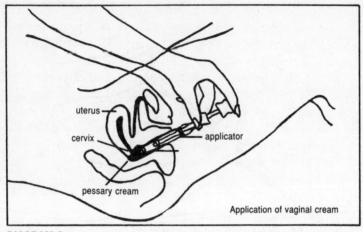

uterus

cervix

applicator

pessary cream

Application of vaginal cream

DIAGRAM 8a

testosterone implant. Three weeks later her blood test showed normal levels of oestrogen and testosterone and Janet was relieved of her symptoms that were supposedly "all in her mind".

Some of the world's foremost experts on the menopause use hormone implants as first-line therapy in menopausal women who complain of fatigue, depression or loss of libido[5]. Oestradiol implants have been shown to increase bone density and can be used to prevent osteoporosis. Psychological and sexual problems occurring after the menopause may be greatly helped by taking the male hormone testosterone. Generally, it is only necessary for a few months. **Testosterone does not work well in tablet form and an implant or intra-muscular injection of natural testosterone provides an ideal alternative**[6]. Testosterone implants and/or injections generally produce a feeling of mental, physical and sexual wellbeing and most women are very happy with their effects. It is only fair to warn any woman considering a testosterone implant that it may cause a slight increase in facial hair or pimples but this decreases when the dose of testosterone is reduced or left off in subsequent implants of oestrogen. If the dose of testosterone implant is kept at 50mg every six to twelve months, it is highly unlikely that undesirable side effects such as facial hair, acne, voice changes or increased cholesterol will occur.

It is important that your suitability for and dosage of oestrogen implant is carefully considered as, once inserted, the implants are difficult to remove in case of overdose or side effects. If side effects occur, they are usually confined to tender breasts or an increase in the heaviness of menstrual bleeding but the latter can usually be controlled by increasing the dose of progesterone.

In a small percentage of women the higher dose oestrogen implants (greater than 50mg) can produce very heavy periods which can be dangerous and frightening as this bleeding may be difficult to stop. This is more likely in women with a past history of heavy periods, an enlarged uterus or fibroids. Some doctors will only use oestrogen implants in women who have had a hysterectomy because of the chance of inducing heavy periods. Oestrogen and testosterone implants are very effective for younger women who have had their uterus and ovaries surgically removed.

In some women (3–8%), the implants may only be effective temporarily and such women find themselves requiring implants at increasingly shorter intervals, even though their blood tests show very high levels of oestrogen. This type of addictive reaction is called tachyphylaxis and it seems in this type of woman they cannot get enough oestrogen. This is not good as it is not natural for the body to have very high levels of oestrogen continually, mainly because it could theoretically increase the risk of breast or uterine cancer. Such women who are addicted to high levels of oestrogen should be transfered to smaller dose implants or oestrogen patches. They will also benefit greatly by taking supplements of Evening Primrose Oil, 4 grams daily, antioxidant vitamins, Vitamin B6, 200mg daily, and a vitamin B complex. This is because very high levels of oestrogen may induce nutritional deficiencies and imbalances in the body.

A safe and reasonable level of oestrogen in the body is 300–500pmol/L as determined by a blood test.

Towards the end of the life of your implant you should have a blood test to check your oestrogen and Follicle Stimulating Hormone (FSH) levels so that another implant can be inserted before oestrogen deficiency returns.

CHAPTER 9

MOST ASKED QUESTIONS ABOUT HORMONE REPLACEMENT THERAPY

Should Every Women Take HRT?

When one looks at the advantages and powerful influence of HRT, it is tempting for doctors to believe that all women should have oestrogen for menopause. But each woman is different, some have no symptoms and are not at risk of cardiovascular disease or osteoporosis and for such women HRT is not medically necessary. But it is the right of every woman to be examined and tested and if found to be at risk she should be offered HRT as an option.

How Long Should I Take HRT?

Around 40% of women still complain of symptoms due to oestrogen deficiency 10 years after their menopause started. Thus, they may still be troubled with hot flushes, vaginal dryness, sweating and lack of sexuality. Such symptoms last for a variable period of time and thus the duration of oestrogen replacement therapy will vary according to the need of the individual woman to control these symptoms. To prevent osteoporosis we need to give oestrogen replacement therapy for 15 to 20 years.

Taking oestrogen protects your bones against calcium loss and your heart and blood vessels against disease but this protection ceases quickly if oestrogen is stopped. The logical conclusion is that ideally you should stay on oestrogen for life, provided you feel well and receive regular check-ups from your doctor. Furthermore, it is never too late to begin HRT and women can still benefit by starting in their 60s and 70s; the notorious actress, Mae West took HRT way into her 80s!

Ultimately, the length of time you take HRT should be your informed choice and you will need to read all of this book and communicate with your doctor before you decide what is right for you.

SIDE EFFECT	SUGGESTION
Breast swelling and tenderness, heavy menstrual bleeding, period pains	Reduce oestrogen dosage and perhaps increase progestagen dosage. Primrose Oil 3gms daily
Increase in blood pressure, fluid retention, bloating, weight gain, aching legs	Reduce oestrogen dosage or change to a non-oral form of oestrogen such as an oestrogen patch or implant
Migraine, headaches, nausea or vomiting	Change to a non-oral form of oestrogen such as patches or implants. Begin with a small dose oestrogen patch or implant
Inability to tolerate menstrual bleeding	Give both oestrogen and progesterone continuously. Consider endometrial ablation
Depression, irritability, mood changes, loss of sex drive	Change to a non-oral form of oestrogen such as oestrogen implants, patches or injections. May need to add testosterone injections or implants often for initial 3 to 12 months only
Facial pigmentation (chloasma)	Reduce oestrogen dosage, change to oestrogen patch or implant. Avoid SUNLIGHT on face, wear hat and sunblock lotion
Premenstrual symptoms (e.g. depression/irritability) during progestagen therapy	Reduce progestagen dose (e.g., to 2.5 mg Provera daily) or change to progesterone injections (Proluton Depot), or Duphaston. Take the progesterone less often—say every 2 or 3 months
Taking HRT and still suffering from oestrogen deficiency symptoms. See oestrogen deficiency score chart Page 25	Have a blood test to check your blood level of oestradiol. If on the low side, increase your tablets or add or change to oestrogen implant, patches or injections. For a dry vagina add oestrogen cream
Large varicose veins or worsening of varicose veins	Reduce oestrogen dose or change to oestrogen patches

TABLE 8

FOOTNOTE: Too much oestrogen causes sore breasts, nausea, fluid retention. Too much progesterone may cause premenstrual syndrome and weight gain.

What Can I Do If I Get Side Effects From HRT?

Usually side effects from HRT are minor and can be overcome by trying smaller doses of hormones or taking a different form of HRT (see Table 8). Rarely, high doses of the oral forms of HRT can cause clots (thrombosis) to form in the circulation and this may produce pain and swelling in the legs, a disturbance of vision, speech, sensation or weakness of the limbs. I emphasise that this is rare and if it occurs you should immediately cease HRT and consult your doctor. Women more prone to such side effects are those with obesity, high blood pressure, varicose veins, a past history of blood clots or strokes, or those who smoke. The oestrogen patches are safe in such high risk women. Some women on HRT complain of a mild to moderate weight gain. This is because HRT may cause a slight increase in appetite and fluid retention. This weight gain can be avoided by reducing the dose of HRT, avoiding masculine progesterones, reducing saturated fats in the diet and regular exercise.

Presently because of side effects fewer than 50% of women who start on HRT will continue with treatment for more than a few months. To prevent osteoporosis HRT must be taken for fifteen to twenty years, if not for life. The reason why many women give up HRT is because they get annoying side effects. I have designed a table to help you and your doctor work out some practical solutions and alternatives if you run into problems with HRT. Remember, patience is a virtue!

Side effects can be minimised by starting with small doses of natural hormones and, if necessary, gradually increasing these until you feel relieved of your symptoms. Your doctor may need to adjust the dose and way of giving you HRT several times to find a programme of HRT to suit you as an individual and to avoid annoying side effects.

Does HRT Cause Weight Gain?

In my experience approximately one in three women who start hormone replacement therapy (HRT) at the menopause will gain a significant amount of weight. This is usually just over 2 kg (4–5lb) but it can occasionally be much more. This tendency can be avoided by asking your doctor to give you the natural brands of oestrogen and progesterone, instead of the synthetic brands of these hormones. Quite a few menopausal ladies find that they need to reduce their dosage of hormone replacement therapy or, failing that, take their hormone replacement therapy in the form of the oestrogen patch instead of tablets, to avoid gaining weight.

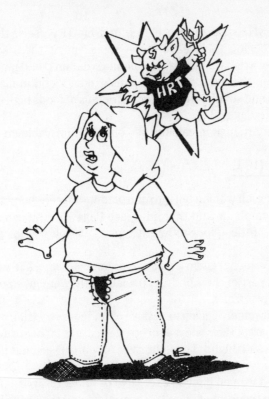

Generally speaking, heavier women require a smaller dose of hormone replacement therapy than lightweight or thin women. They may need to take a smaller amount of progesterone, either by breaking the tablet in half or quarters or by taking it for a shorter time in each calendar month. The natural progesterone called Dydrogesterone (Duphaston) is less likely to put on weight than are the other brands of progesterone — namely, Primolut and Provera. Unfortunately, Duphaston is more expensive, but your private health fund may cover the cost.

The oestrogen patch is available under the brand of Estraderm and comes in three strengths — Estraderm 100, Estraderm 50 and Estraderm 25.

The smaller doses in the weaker oestrogen patches, for example, Estraderm 50 and/or 25 are most unlikely to cause weight gain. Generally speaking, it is possible by reducing the doses of oestrogen and progesterone in your hormone replacement therapy, to avoid any significant weight gain.

If, despite all these measures, hormone replacement therapy still causes unwanted weight gain, you may decide to give it away altogether, but check with your doctor first as you may be losing the great advantages that oestrogen replacement therapy has for your skeleton and blood vessels. If after all consideration you decide to give hormone replacement therapy away, I suggest you consume a diet that is high in calcium, vitamin D and natural food sources of oestrogen. Natural plant oestrogens can be found in many foods such as green beans and soya beans and for full details of foods high in natural plant oestrogens, see Page 88.

To find foods that are high in calcium see our Calcium Table on Page 98.

Body Types and HRT

Generally speaking, all women fall into one of four different body shapes — android, gynaeoid, lymphatic and thyroid — see Page 75. You can also be a combination of two of these four different types, but you will fall predominantly into one type.

Android-shaped women if given excessive or unnecessary HRT will put on weight in the upper part of their body, especially if they are given excessive progesterone or testosterone.

Gynaeoid-shaped women if given excessive or unnecessary HRT will put on weight in the lower part of their body, as oestrogen causes fat deposition in the pelvic area, buttocks and thighs. Thus, this type of woman becomes more pear shaped.

Lymphatic-shaped women if given excessive or unnecessary HRT will put on weight all over, in the form of an extra layer of fat and they will also retain fluid in their limbs.

Thyroid-shaped women gain weight less easily than the other body shapes — nonetheless they can gain weight in their abdomen and thighs if given an excessive dose of HRT. Generally speaking thin thyroid types of women tolerate higher doses of HRT without significant weight gain.

If you have worked with your doctor to find the correct dose of HRT and yet still find yourself gaining weight and don't know why, I advise you to investigate your diet more thoroughly. You may be consuming excess calories or a diet that is wrong for your particular body shape. Each of the four body shapes has a different metabolism and hormonal balance and you will lose weight most effectively if you follow a scientifically balanced diet and food combinations to match your body shape. This unique weight loss diet is called the Body Shaping Diet. It is available under this title as a book which lists step-by-step meal plans and recipes formulated for each of the four body shapes to achieve effective weight loss and body shaping.

BODY TYPES

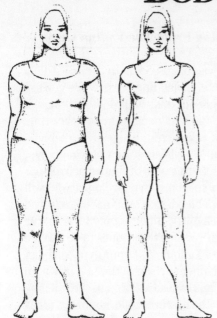

Android body shape (left) overweight, (right) ideal weight

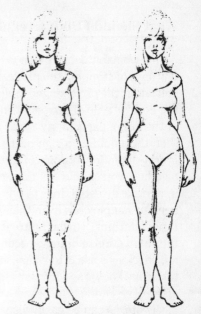

Gynaeoid body shape (left) overweight, (right) ideal weight

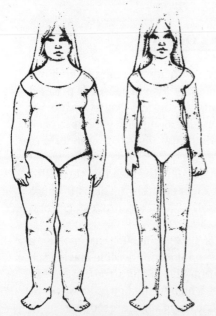

Lymphatic body shape (left) overweight, (right) ideal weight

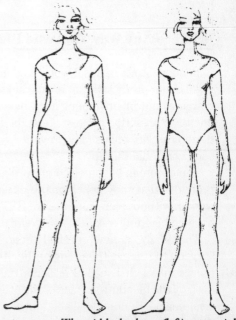

Thyroid body shape (left) overweight, (right) ideal weight

What Should I Do If Irregular Bleeding From The Vagina Occurs?

In a woman taking HRT it is normal for vaginal bleeding to occur within a few days of stopping the progestagen tablets. If bleeding starts while you are still taking the progestagen tablets you may need to ask your doctor to change the dose or type of progestagen tablets. If bleeding occurs at any other time of the cycle, particularly when you are not taking your progestagen tablets, then this could be a sign of disease in your uterus such as a uterine polyp, uterine infection, fibroids or uterine cancer. In this type of abnormal irregular bleeding, you should ask for a referral to a specialist gynaecologist who will undertake investigations to find the cause of bleeding. The gynaecologist will need to sample cells from the entire surface of the inner lining of the uterus (endometrium), so that no areas are missed. Suitable techniques to do this are the vabra curette or a gynoscan. A newer technique that your gynaecologist may decide to use is to visualise the entire inner surface of the uterus with a telescope known as a hysteroscope that is gently passed through the opening of the cervix under a local anaesthetic. With the hysteroscope, abnormal areas of the uterus can be easily visualised, then sampled with a currette and sent to a laboratory for testing. Once this has been done you can feel reassured that your irregular bleeding is not a sign of disease and you may continue with your HRT.

Is There Any Way To Avoid Bleeding On HRT?

Some postmenopausal women cannot cope with any bleeding, even if it is regular and predictable, at an age in life when they wish to be free of periods, tampons and inconvenient napkins and pads. If you feel like this ask your doctor to prescribe progestagen tablets every day along with your oestrogen therapy as this will usually prevent any bleeding after three to four months of such continual therapy.

Some women become so annoyed and fatigued by the bleeding their HRT produces that they consider the option of a hysterectomy! This is because women without a uterus can take HRT by itself without any progestagen and have no bleeding at all.

Thankfully, a new surgical technique is now available that enables a surgeon to remove the lining of the uterus (endometrium) while leaving the uterus intact. It is called endometrial ablation and enables the surgeon to destroy the bleeding surface of the uterus with high frequency radio waves or laser beams. Endometrial ablation can be done using a hysteroscope through the cervix so that no cutting or stitches are required and thus post-operative discomfort, pain and time off work are minimal.

The success of endometrial ablation varies so that afterwards you may find that you have no further bleeding or that the amount of bleeding is reduced to varying degrees. For best results go to a gynaecologist who has a lot of experience in performing hysteroscopy and endometrial ablations.

After an endometrial ablation, it is still necessary to take some progester-one tablets every month, even though your menstrual bleeding will be much less or non-existent.

Are There Any Reasons Why I Can't Take Oestrogen?

Modern-day natural HRT is very flexible and safe and only a minority of women are told by their doctors that they should avoid it. If you suffer with the following problems you will generally be advised never to take oestrogen:

1. Oestrogen-dependent cancers such as cancer of the breast or uterine lining (endometrium).
2. Severe liver disease such as cirrhosis.

Doctors are generally reluctant to give oestrogen to women who have previously been treated for uterine cancer because of a possible stimulation to the distant spread of the cancer. However, if the cancer had been detected in the early stages and had been of the less aggressive type on pathological testing and the patient had remained cancer-free for at least two years, some doctors may feel it safe to prescribe oestrogen in small doses to a patient who complains of severe oestrogen deficiency.

Some women who have been successfully treated for breast cancer find that they are unable to tolerate a complete lack of sex hormones in their body and HRT programmes using very small doses of oestrogen and larger doses of progesterone can be worked out for them. They may choose to take this type of HRT after weighing up all pros and cons with their cancer specialist. If the cancer has been completely removed and the lymph glands in the armpits are free of cancer, then there is a 75% chance of a complete cure and as far as we know giving HRT may not dramatically change things. A woman may live another twenty to thirty years after successful treatment for breast cancer and may not want to run the increased risk of bone fractures or heart attacks that could occur without oestrogen.

There are several other medical problems that would make a doctor very careful about giving you oestrogen. They are not, however, absolute reasons that you cannot take HRT. You may indeed, but extra vigilance and care is required. These medical problems are:

- Recent or severe blood clots or thrombosis—the statistical risk of blood clots is not increased by HRT, but if there is a past history of clots many doctors prefer to use the oestrogen patches, as they are the safest way of giving HRT.
- Mild liver disease.
- Severe blood pressure that is difficult to control with drugs.
- Fibroids or endometriosis—if HRT is given, pain and irregular bleeding can be a problem and surgical treatment may be required.
- Gall bladder disease—this may be aggravated by HRT.
- Large, tender, very lumpy breasts (mastopathy).
- Systemic lupus erythematosus.

If you feel that oestrogen replacement therapy is too dangerous for you, please refer to Page 88 and find out how you can obtain small amounts of natural plant oestrogen safely through foods.

Will HRT Increase My Risk Of Cancer?

If one analyses all the published literature and clinical trials to date, it can be concluded that generally speaking death rates from all cancers are not increased by the correct use of HRT. However, very long-term studies are not available and it will be several decades before the real effect of natural HRT on the promotion or reduction of different cancers will be known.

Cancer of the Uterine Lining (Endometrium)

Presently, it appears that HRT reduces the risk of this cancer as well as ovarian cancer, perhaps by up to 40% compared to women not using HRT. This only applies if progesterone is given for at least 12–14 days of every monthly cycle.

Breast Cancer

Many women are reluctant to take HRT fearing that it will increase their chances of breast cancer. This remains a complicated and controversial issue, especially as we are talking about the most common cancer in western women. Statistics show that breast cancer will affect one in every fifteen women by the age of 75 and one in eight women with a family history of this disease. Some of these cancers have oestrogen receptors and there is the possibility that these may be promoted by oestrogen therapy. The risk of breast cancer peaks in your 50s and 60s and continues to rise progressively throughout life and so at this time one certainly does not want to take a substance that may further increase this risk. Risk factors for breast cancer include lack of childbirth, first childbirth after thirty, obesity, early puberty, family history of breast cancer and a late menopause. A common feature in these factors is prolonged and constant exposure to oestrogen from the ovaries. Women whose diets are high in fat and low in fibre have higher blood levels of oestrogen than women on low-fat, high-fibre diets. Women on high-fat, low-fibre diets have a much higher incidence of breast cancer and so it seems that we have yet another possible link between oestrogen and breast cancer.

Notwithstanding these theoretical considerations, of nearly 30 studies examining the relationship between oestrogen replacement and breast cancer, the majority have failed to indicate a definitive for or against[8]. Individually, these studies have found either a small decrease or small increase in the future incidence of breast cancer in users of HRT. A widely publicised 1989 Swedish study linked oestrogen with a slightly increased risk of breast cancer after six or more years of use. However, their conclusions were premature as they only followed up these women for an average duration of 5.7 years, when it is known that most breast cancers take seven years to grow large enough for detection. The same Swedish group found that when women using oestrogen developed breast cancer, their survival rate was significantly better than that of women not on oestrogen.

A very useful overview of 23 studies suggested that HRT does not increase or decrease breast cancer[9]. However, the results of studies on long term use of HRT (more than 10 years) counteract this finding and suggest that there may be a small increase in the risk of breast cancer. This increase is in the order of 1.3[18]. This means that if you take oestrogen replacement therapy for more than ten years you may have a 30% increased risk of breast cancer. Although the studies which show this increased risk are only population studies and not rigorously designed scientific trials, they should still make us cautious in prescribing high or prolonged doses of oestrogen replacement therapy to women with a high risk of breast cancer. In such cases, I believe it is wise to use smaller or intermittent doses of oestrogen replacement therapy. The same study found that the risk of breast cancer does not increase until after at least five years of oestrogen replacement therapy and this is reassuring for women who only want to take oestrogen replacement therapy for a short time.

In summary, with HRT of less than five years duration, there is no increase in the incidence of breast cancer.

Incidence may increase after ten to fifteen years of HRT and this increase is in the magnitude of 30%.

Furthermore, while it appears the incidence of breast cancer may increase with long term HRT, women who get this cancer while on HRT are less likely to die from it.

As far as progesterone is concerned we have insufficient data to suggest that it offers any protection against breast cancer in women on oestrogen therapy.

Skin Cancer

Studies suggest that the use of oestrogen has no adverse effect on the subsequent development of malignant melanoma or other skin cancers.

In summary — *It does not appear that properly balanced, natural HRT encourages the development of cancer and any slight increase in the death rate from cancer would be small indeed compared to the reduction in the death rate from osteoporosis, heart disease and stroke in oestrogen users.*

What Are The Hormonal Myths?

TABLE OF MYTHS

MYTH	TRUTH
If I start on HRT can I ever come off it?	Yes, HRT is not addictive.
The menopause can be fully treated with nutritional medicine.	Everyone is an individual and some women require oestrogen replacement therapy.
HRT should be given in the lowest possible dose for the shortest possible time.	In some women HRT should be continued for life.
HRT never causes weight gain.	It can in some women, even if they do not eat more or exercise less. (See Page 72)
HRT increases cancer risk.	Properly balanced HRT reduces cancer risk, except for breast cancer where further long term studies are required.
If HRT brings back my periods can I fall pregnent?	This is impossible as a menopausal women has no eggs left in her ovaries.
I do not need HRT until after my menstrual bleeding ceases.	A deficiency of oestrogen may occur many years before this.
The menopause is short-lived.	It is an epoch with effects lasting until the end of life.

TABLE 9

Will I Become Less Feminine After The Menopause?

The menopausal ovary produces very little oestrogen but continues to make some male hormones. This may cause a hormonal imbalance where a menopausal woman has a relative excess of male hormones.

In some women this may result in an increase in masculine features — more facial hair, thinning of the scalp hair, coarsening of the skin and facial features, shrinkage of the breasts and a slight deepening of the voice.

In most cases this imbalance is easily fixed simply by taking natural oestrogen replacement which will increase your body's female hormones and at the same time reduce the production of male hormones from the ovaries. This will greatly lessen the development of masculine features.

If oestrogen replacement alone is not sufficient to prevent excess facial hair or thinning of the scalp hair it may be necessary to use a special hormone called an "anti-male hormone". The most effective anti-male hormone is called Androcur and its chemical name is cyproterone acetate. Androcur is a remarkable drug that reduces the production and action of male hormones in the body. As well as this it also acts like the female hormone progesterone and can be prescribed along with oestrogen to regulate and balance a menstrual blood flow.

The most effective HRT for a menopausal woman troubled with facial hair and/or balding is a combination of natural oestrogen and Androcur.

If you still have your uterus your doctor can prescribe Androcur for two or three weeks of every calendar month along with oestrogen every day and this will bring on a light menstrual flow. If you have had a hysterectomy you may take oestrogen and Androcur every day (see Table 10).

Androcur has been shown to cure excess facial and body hair in 80% of women after nine to twelve months of use and around one in every two women with balding of the scalp will obtain a regrowth or thickening of the hair after nine to twelve months of taking Androcur.

Pregnancy must be avoided while taking Androcur as it can reduce male sexual development in a foetus.

Because Androcur is a potent anti-male hormone high doses of it may cause a reduction in sex drive, reduced concentration, fatigue and mild depression. Generally, such side effects can be avoided if Androcur is used in a small dosage and once you have noticed an improvement in your skin and scalp hair the dosage can be reduced to about 2.5–5mg daily when side effects should disappear. In the long term the lowest possible dose that can control facial hair should be used and your own doctor can guide you on this. Androcur is available on an authority prescription for women suffering with the effects of excessive male hormones and in such cases is not expensive.

The drug Aldactone, also known as spironolactone is another variety of anti-male hormone, although it is less powerful than Androcur. Some women may find Aldactone is sufficient to control their facial hair, either alone or with natural oestrogen (see Table 10).

What Can I Do If I Have Too Many Male Hormones?

Excessive male hormone activity in your body may produce unsightly facial or body hair, baldness and acne. Thankfully, we can control these annoying things with modern day HRT. See Table 10 to learn about your options.

PROBLEMS	HORMONAL MEASURES	OTHER MEASURES
Excess facial and body hair	1. Natural oestrogen daily plus Androcur 2.5mg to 100mg for 2 or 3 weeks every month. 2. Aldactone 50mg to 200mg daily by itself or with natural oestrogen.	Under the supervision of a beautician Plucking—not recommended Waxing—not for very coarse thick hair Bleaching—for moustache Depilatory creams Shaving—does not increase hair regrowth Electrolysis—for small areas only
Balding	3. Natural oestrogen by itself may be sufficient in mild cases. You will also need progesterone or Androcur if you have a uterus.	Check function of the thyroid gland. Specific nutritional supplements can be very helpful such as: 1. Calcium 1000mg daily. 2. Evening Primrose Oil capsules, 3000mg daily. 3. Zinc chelate 30mg daily. 4. Organic mineral formula 1 daily.
Acne	4. In women unable to take oestrogen Androcur can be taken alone. 5. Cortisone type drug in small dosage e.g. dexamethasone 0.25mg to 0.5mg at night.	1. 'Retin A' cream—is also anti-ageing. 2. Anti-oxidants, Evening Primrose Oil, zinc. 3. WHAS cleansing lotion. 4. WHAS herbal skin peel.

TABLE 10

FOOTNOTE: These are suggested schedules only and your doctor may vary them to suit your particular case.

FOR PRODUCT AVAILABILITY CHART SEE PAGE 133

At What Age Will I Pass Through The Menopause?

While the average age of the menopause is 50 years, some women go through a premature menopause in their 20s, 30s or early 40s, whilst others continue to menstruate up until their late 50s. If menstruation started early in life you are more likely to have a late menopause. Women who have had a hysterectomy, even though they have kept their ovaries, may experience menopause up to four years earlier than the average age. This is because the blood supply to the ovaries may have been decreased after removal of the uterus.

What Should I Know If My Menopause Is Early?

Premature menopause is defined as menopause occurring under the age of 40 years. Often the cause of a premature menopause cannot be determined. However, factors that may play a role are hereditary traits, stress, heavy smoking, poor diet and excessive alcohol consumption and imbalances in your immune system (auto immune diseases). A woman with a premature menopause may have been born with fewer eggs and if they are used at the normal rate, these would soon be depleted. Radiotherapy for pelvic cancer or cancer chemotherapy can quickly destroy a large number of eggs, leaving insufficient to last. Severe infection of the ovaries caused by viruses such as mumps, can also damage large numbers of eggs. In some cases, the ovary goes into a dormant phase and although there may be enough eggs, they refuse to respond. Sometimes this produces a temporary premature menopause and the ovaries occasionally come back into action. Removing the ovaries surgically before the age of 40 years brings on a sudden and severe premature menopause if HRT is not given.

Women with a premature menopause of any cause are at early and increased risk of cardiovascular disease and osteoporosis. To prevent these debilitating diseases, women with a premature menopause should be given HRT *at* the time of their menopause. This will give them adequate protection.

Women who go through a premature menopause frequently experience a whole range of negative emotions such as anger, disbelief, shock, resentment and shame. If you are in this situation it is important that you receive counselling from a sympathetic doctor because if you bottle up such negative emotions, you may find yourself feeling very depressed.

If you have a very early menopause — say under the age of 30 years, you may find it difficult to relate to information on menopause that has been designed for 50-year-old women and thus find yourself becoming increasingly isolated. However, if you can find an understanding doctor, then these negative feelings will not last. It is important to understand that menopause is not synonymous with old age, it merely means that your ovaries have exhausted their supply of eggs quicker than normal.

A premature menopause if properly treated will not cause you to age more quickly, change your personality or mental ability and indeed to all of your friends and family you will appear just the same as before menopause.

When it comes to your sex life, adequate HRT should enable you to feel and act just as sexy as ever. You may need a larger dose or different form of HRT than a woman of 50 or 60 and for details concerning HRT and sex, turn to Page 110.

If I Have A Premature Menopause Can I Have Children?

Generally, by the time a premature menopause is diagnosed, fertility is very low and it may often be too late to try and stimulate ovulation with fertility drugs. Many of these women have previously adopted children and recently the option of obtaining a donor egg or embryo has become possible. Donor eggs and embryos enable women who do not have a living supply of their own eggs to have the chance of a lifetime. Normally, the chosen donor would be a close relative and she too must take part in an in vitro fertilisation (IVF) programme, where her ovaries are hyper-stimulated to produce a crop of premium eggs. Once collected, the donor eggs are fertilised in a test tube (in vitro) with the husband's sperm. The resulting embryo is then implanted into the menopausal woman's uterus which has been suitably prepared with hormones. If a relative is unavailable, spare donor eggs or embryos from an unrelated person who is going through the IVF programme may be available. The egg and embryo donor programme has been fairly successful, with a 25% to 40% chance of a normal pregnancy.

Yes, it is amazing to think that egg donation offers menopausal women of any age the possibility to fall pregnant and have a baby. I wonder if we shall see many women in their 50s and 60s having maternal urges?

At The End Of The Day, Is HRT Really Safe?

Thus far our experience using HRT in large numbers of women has produced some interesting statistics. If we look at all the major studies done so far and try to be as honest, if not a little pessimistic, as we can be, the results come out in favour of taking HRT, as its benefits outweigh its risks. For example, if we took 100,000 women and gave them oestrogen replacement therapy, there would be 38 who get breast cancer, however 366 of these women would be saved from stroke, heart disease and osteoporotic fractures[11]. In other words we save more lives than we lose by using long term HRT. Diagram 9 (below) shows this diagrammatically.

But still today the case for universally treating all menopausal women with HRT remains controversial, especially as this would include treating women with no symptoms and no risk factors for osteoporosis or cardiovascular disease.

It is easy to understand why many menopausal women feel confused, when controversy and disagreement exists amongst the medical profession and some women feel that they don't want to be part of a generation of hormone guinea pigs. In one hundred years from now we will have more conclusive evidence if giving HRT saves lives but, in the meantime, you may not want to wait so long!

Nothing in life can promise to be perfect and generally speaking today's woman seeks the best compromise or balance between all her options.

At the end of the day, it is you who must decide what the best option for your individual lifestyle and long term health requirements is.

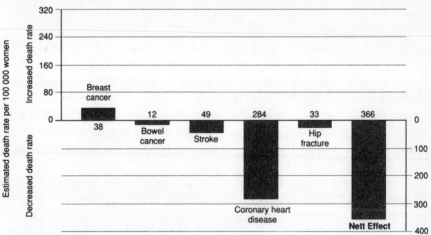

DIAGRAM 9 OESTROGEN AND DEATH RATES

Whether you decide to take HRT or use the nutritional therapies described in Chapters 10 and 11, you should see your doctor, at least annually, for the rest of your life because your requirements for therapy often change over the years.

CHAPTER 10

CAN NATUROPATHIC MEDICINE HELP WITH YOUR MENOPAUSE?

This chapter was written jointly by Dr Sandra Cabot and Deborah Cooper, a naturopath and herbalist specialising in women's health who has a practice in Sydney.

For 20 years I have prescribed various combinations of vitamins, minerals, essential fatty acids and herbs in addition to orthodox medicines, to aid the achievement of optimum wellbeing during the menopausal years. The tremendous difference these nutritional supplements can make never ceases to amaze me and I firmly believe that they are worth the extra effort and expense.

A menopausal woman may not be able to take oestrogen replacement therapy because of certain medical problems such as breast cancer, liver disease or blood clots. Others choose to avoid hormone replacement for personal or philosophical reasons and some actually feel better without hormones. In such cases naturopathic medicine can be extremely helpful, reducing hot flushes, dryness and wrinkling of the skin, anxiety and stress and also improving the function of the immune system. Whether you take HRT or not, naturopathic supplements can be used to great advantage. Study our handy reference Table 11 to see how they may help you.

CAN NATUROPATHIC MEDICINE HELP WITH YOUR MENOPAUSE?

PROBLEM	STRATEGY
Hot flushes, sweating	Increase water intake to 2 litres daily. Vitamin E 500iu, once or twice daily. Evening Primrose Oil 3000mg daily. Herbs Sarsaparilla and Don Quai.
Dry itchy skin and dry vagina	Evening Primrose Oil 3000mg daily. Increase water intake to 2 litres daily. Anti-oxidants such as vitamins A, C, E, Betacarotene, Selenium.
Fatigue, poor memory and reduced mental efficiency	Ginseng capsules 500mg, 3 times daily. Ginkgo Biloba tablets 600mg, 3 times daily. High potency B complex tablets, 1 daily.
Rapid ageing of the skin, thinning of hair, brittle nails	Mineral Complex 2 daily. Evening Primrose Oil 3000mg daily, or in severe cases, a very concentrated source of all essential fatty acids from evening primrose oil, borage oil and fish oil. Bianca's Collagen and Elastin Cream (micronised) and Cell Repairer cream. Antioxidants tablets, 2 daily.
Anxiety, irritability, insomnia	The gentle sedative herbs, passion flower, valerian, lime flowers, oats and scullcap, Amino Acid complex. High potency vitamin B complex tablets.
Muscle and joint aches and pains, deterioration of the bones and joints	Evening Primrose Oil and fish oil, 4 capsules daily. Antioxidant tablets, 1 or 2 daily. Organic Mineral Complex, 2 daily.

TABLE 11

FOR PRODUCT AVAILABILITY CHART SEE PAGE 133

NATURAL PLANT OESTROGENS

Over 300 different plants contain oestrogenic substances. Although these are only weak oestrogens and are present in tiny quantities, if the foods they are found in are consumed regularly they can exert a mild oestrogenic effect in humans [13&14].

Plant oestrogens are found in bourbon, whisky, gin, pernot, ouzo and beer. These oestrogens are partly responsible for the breast development seen in alcoholic males, as their damaged livers are unable to break down and inactivate the oestrogens found in alcohol. By the way, I don't recommend you try to increase your oestrogen levels by drinking alcohol! Alfalfa contains the plant oestrogen called coumestrol and may cause infertility in animals grazing on large pastures of alfalfa grasses. Of all the plant oestrogens coumestrol is the most potent, but is 200 times weaker than human oestrogens. The herb red clover contains coumestrol and can be taken in the form of a herbal tea or you can make fresh sprouts from red clover seeds. As some types of red clover are poisonous, it is best to obtain supplies from a herbalist or reputable health food store. Soya beans, soya sprouts and linseed meal (crushed seeds), are excellent sources of natural oestrogens, protein and essential fatty acids. They are definitely anti-ageing foods for menopausal women. For guidance in foods and herbs containing plant oestrogens see Table below.

FOODS CONTAINING NATURAL OESTROGENS ARE:			
linseed	garlic	green beans	red beans
pumpkin	split peas	marrow	cow pea
olives	olive oil	soya bean	bakers' yeast
parsley	chick peas	rhubarb	cherry
corn	oats	barley	rye
wheat	rice	peas	sesame
liquorice	french beans	clover	red clover
apple	fennel	alfalfa	aniseed
hops	sage	corn oil	sunflower
carrots	beetroot	plum	squash
cabbage	soya sprouts	potato	

TABLE 12

These foods are high in not only oestrogens, but also vitamins, minerals, fibre and essential fatty acids and are low in saturated fat. Thus there are many good reasons to consume them on a regular basis.

The natural plant oestrogens in the foods contained in Table 12 are a useful and safe form of oestrogen supplementation for women who are unable to take oestrogen replacement therapy because of a past history of breast or uterine cancer or for women not wanting to take larger doses of hormones in conventional forms.

Because these plant oestrogens are so weak they are safe and will not produce the side effects sometimes seen with conventional forms of HRT. If you want to boost your oestrogen levels, I suggest you eat approximately two cups daily of foods from Table 12. For example, two cups of mixed sprouts, parsley, soya beans, legumes, fennel, along with a wide selection of fresh vegetables. Make sure you vary your sources of plant oestrogens by using different foods from the Table to make up your two cups worth of oestrogenic foods each day.

HERBS FOR MENOPAUSE

There are many herbs that contain plant oestrogens or act as stimulants in the production of your natural hormones. These herbs can "bridge the gap" from when your ovaries cease their function and when your adrenal glands take over by producing a different form of oestrogen called "oestrone".

Oestrone is not as powerful as the ovaries' oestrogen called oestradiol, however it is often enough to reduce your symptoms during this transition period.

Many women prefer the process of menopause to be a natural one. There are also women who are unable to take HRT. The good news for these women is that they do have an alternative.

Listed below are herbs suitable for menopause with a brief overview of their actions, as well as information on their preparation and dosage. These herbs can be purchased from health food outlets or from a herbalist.

I encourage you to try the herbal teas, however some of you may need to consult with a qualified herbalist who will dispense your herbs and advise according to your individual requirements.

SALVIA OFFICINALIS - Sage
(Fresh or dried leaves)
This herb has many medicinal properties and is very useful during meno-

pause for the treatment of hot flushes. Sage reduces excessive sweating and it contains plant oestrogens. You will find sage particularly useful in eliminating night sweats.

GLYCORRHIZA GABRA - Licorice
(Dried root and rhizome)

Licorice is a powerful adrenal stimulant and is a wonderful oestrogenic herb. For this reason it is a very useful herb at menopause.

However, care must be taken not to drink this tea too often. Large doses can deplete potassium in your body and elevate blood pressure, so take care if you are hypertensive. On the other hand, if you suffer from low blood pressure then this herb will be useful in correcting this problem.

It is a pleasant tasting tea that can be combined with other herbal teas to improve their flavour. We recommend 1 to 2 cups of licorice herbal tea daily for hot flushes.

CIMICIFUGA RACEMOSA - Black Cohosh
(Dried root and rhizome)

A good oestrogenic herb that acts specifically on the uterus to reduce cramps and congestion. This herb contains two anti-rheumatic agents and is excellent for relieving muscular pain and cramping.

ALETRIS FARINOSA - True Unicorn Root
(Dried root and rhizome)

This oestrogenic herb will tonify the female genital organs. It is a bitter herb that is also useful for indigestion and it has a mild sedative action.

CHAMAELIRIUM LUTEUM - False Unicorn Root
(Dried root and rhizome)

This plant is an oestrogen regulator. It has a direct action on the uterus and ovaries and is considered to be a corrective herb for women.

It is helpful in the herbal treatment of ovarian cysts.

DIOSCOREA VILLOSA - Wild Yam
(Dried root and rhizome)

Wild yam is a powerful oestrogenic herb used by women worldwide. It has a good anti-inflammatory action and will give relief from menopausal arthritis.

CAPSELLA BURSA - Shepherd's Purse
(Dried flowering plant; fresh plant)

Shepherd's purse is a pituitary regulator with androgenic properties. One of its primary functions is its ability to normalise progesterone levels.

If you are moving into menopause and have been experiencing excessive, irregular bleeding or spotting, then drinking this tea will help to regulate and increase the length of your menstrual cycle until your natural cessation of menses.

TRIFOLIUM PRATENSE - Red Clover
(Dried flower heads; fresh plant)

Red clover contains a plant oestrogen called coumestrol and one of its medicinal actions is to stimulate the ovaries. It is a good "alkalinising" herb described in herbals as an alterative herb, which means "to restore healthy body functions".

SMILAX - Sarsparilla
(Dried root and rhizome)

Sarsparilla is another alterative herb and stimulates testosterone production and therefore improves a flagging libido.

SAW PALMETTO
(Dried fruit)

This herb is beneficial in the treatment of urinary incontinence and prolapse.

Dryness and a lack of tone in the bladder often leads to bladder irritation and weakness which is reduced by saw palmetto.

TARAXACUM OFFICINALE - Dandelion
(Dried root)

Dandelion is a wonderful herb for the liver. Your liver is under extra stress when hormones are out of balance and drinking dandelion root beverage will be beneficial.

RUBUS IDAEUS - Raspberry Leaf
(Fresh or dried leaves and fruit)

Raspberry is an astringent and oestrogenic herb. It has a direct action on the uterine muscles and therefore will help to tone weakened muscles and will assist in correcting prolapse.

VITEX AGNUS CASTUS - Chaste Tree
(Dried fruit)
   This herb is a hormone balancer that is used to alleviate depression at menopause.

TURNERA DIFFUSA - Damiana
(Dried leaves)
   A great herb for menopause because it is a pituitary regulator and antidepressant. It is an aphrodisiac and is of benefit in sexual debility. It should not be taken too frequently or it may irritate the lining of your urinary tract; we recommend 2 or 3 times per week.

HYPERICUM - St John's Wort
(Fresh or dried flowering plant)
   This herb is a mild sedative that is specific for anxiety states.

SENECIO AUREAS - Life Root
(Dried plant)
   Life root is a uterine tonic that contains plant oestrogens. It will re-establish emotional and vascular stability and help to eliminate hot flushes.

Preparation of Herbal Teas

   The flowers and leaves of herbs are prepared by making a tea. Allow 15g of the dried herb to 250ml of boiled water. Prepare the tea in a glass or ceramic teapot which has a tight fitting lid. Let the "infusion" steep for 10–15 minutes, strain and drink.

   If you are using the dried root, seeds or woody parts of a plant then you will need to make a "decoction". This is made by adding 15g of the dried herb to 250ml of cold water in a glass or enamel saucepan. Let the mixture soak for 10 minutes and then cover and bring to the boil. Reduce heat and simmer for 15 minutes. Remove from the heat and let it steep for a further 10 minutes. Strain and drink warm.

   DOSAGE — A cupful should be taken warm, not hot, 3 times a day.

STRATEGIES FOR HEALTHY BLOOD VESSELS

Heart and blood vessel disease is the number one killer of women in westernised societies, claiming twice as many lives as cancer. After menopause, women are at significant risk of heart and blood vessel disease. Although these diseases attack women later than men, this should not stop women looking at ways to decrease their risk until later in life. Survival rates after heart attacks are less in women than men, for every age group.

Let us take a look at some of the nutritional strategies we can use to decrease our risk of cardiovascular disease.

These good nutritional habits will also reduce your risk of cancer and obesity.

MINIMISE FATS

Reducing fats in your diet will reduce your risk of heart disease and cancer.

Fats and oils are extremely high in calories and if excessive amounts are eaten they will slow down your metabolic rate, stop you losing weight and contribute to obesity.

Many fats can be reduced in your diet simply by changing habits and cooking techniques. A quick way to lessen the amount of fats in your diet is to stop buying processed foods such as packaged biscuits, cakes, pastries or fried foods which are high in fat. Also when you are selecting a breakfast cereal, take the time to read the product information on the packaging. You may be surprised to find that some popular brands have very high levels of fat, salt and sugar. Good low-fat alternatives to processed breakfast cereals are oatmeal porridge, barley, brown rice or natural unsweetened muesli.

You can make yourself an excellent mixture called LSA that can be added to your breakfast cereal.

LSA = Linseeds (3 parts) sunflower seeds (2 parts) almonds (1 part)

Mix and grind together into a fine meal. LSA is an excellent concentrated source of omega 6 essential fatty acids, fibre, protein, calcium, selenium, vitamins E, A and B. You can also purchase LSA from a health food store; it must be fresh and stored in the refrigerator.

Start making healthy choices and feel the benefits.

TYPES OF FAT
Saturated Fats

These fats are the most important ones to reduce as excessive amounts can lead to obesity, clogged arteries, and an increased risk of cancer of the breast, ovaries, uterus and bowel. The best way to identify a saturated fat is that it is solid at room temperature. Examples of saturated fats are the fats found in beef, pork, lamb, poultry, full cream milk, cream, cheese, ice cream, chocolate, ghee, butter, copha, dripping, suet, lard, coconut and palm oils. I am not suggesting that you avoid these foods completely, but make sure that you remove *all* the fat from meat and the skin from chicken and use low-fat dairy products. You may safely eat red meat 3–4 times per week, provided you remove all fat. Never fry red meat or chicken, grill these meats or use them in casseroles and stews. Eggs contain cholesterol but may be eaten in moderation, 4 eggs per week being advisable as they are an excellent source of sulphur containing amino acids. Boil or poach your eggs, never fry them as when fried, eggs produce dangerous oxycholesterol.

Processed or delicatessan meats, such as fritz, smoked or pressed ham, salami, cabanossi, etc., are not healthy to eat as they are loaded with saturated fats and, as they are not fresh, their fats may become rancid. Rancid fats are highly oxidised and will generate free radicals in your body that attack your blood vessels and body cells.

Cholesterol

Cholesterol is a pearly fatlike substance that is produced in your liver. It cannot dissolve in water or blood and is transported in your body by lipoproteins. High-density lipoproteins are scavengers and help to clean up cholesterol and carry it back to the liver to be reused or broken down. Lipoproteins are not found in foods but are manufactured by the liver. You can increase the beneficial high-density lipoproteins by exercising regularly, reducing saturated fats in the diet, maintaining a healthy weight and not smoking. Your body can produce all the cholesterol you need without the need for added dietary cholesterol. If your dietary cholesterol is high it may end up being deposited on the walls of your arteries leading to hardening and blockage of the arteries. By having low dietary cholesterol your need for high-density lipoproteins is also low.

Generally, it is ideal to have a blood cholesterol level of between 2.6 and 5.5 mmol/L and in some people elevated blood cholesterol may increase the risk of heart disease. Cholesterol is found in saturated fats. Foods rich in saturated fats are all land animal products such as fatty meats, pre-served meats, full-cream dairy foods, shellfish, coconut and palm oil. Reducing dietary saturated fat is only one of the methods of reducing cholesterol levels. You must also increase foods which will help to lower cholesterol. Such foods are oily fish, vitamin C rich foods (citrus fruits, watermelon, cabbage, fresh green leafy vegetables, kiwi fruits, peppers and strawberries), garlic, onion and foods containing soluble fibre. Soluble fibre dissolves easily in water and is found in the gums, pectin and mucilages of plant fibre. Such soluble fibre is found in legumes, cereals, grains, oatbran, fruits and vegetables. Soluble fibre protects us against gall stones, ulcerative colitis, high blood pressure, high blood cholesterol and diabetes.

Unsaturated Fats
These are liquid or soft at room temperature. Examples are fish oils, soft margarines, olive, linseed, canola, grapeseed, peanut, corn, safflower, sesame, soybean and sunflower oils. These oils are a combination of mono-unsaturated and polyunsaturated oils. The best choices of these oils are olive, canola, or linseed. This is because these oils contain mono-unsaturated oils. Research has shown that these oils can be beneficial to the health of our arteries[15]. Mediterranean people consume these oils regularly and have very low rates of heart disease.

Try to obtain *cold pressed* vegetable and seed oils as none of these fats and oils are healthy if we subject them to heat processing or if we fry food in them. Animal fats and vegetable oils when they are heated at high temperatures form chemicals which attack and destroy blood vessel walls.

If you use butter or margarine on your bread and crackers, use them only in moderation. Butter is a natural product, but is high in cholesterol and calories. Margarine is a synthetic product and many brands contain excessive chemicals to make them look and taste like butter. Many margarines contain Cis and trans-fatty acids which are formed during the hydrogenation process used during the manufacture of margarine and shortening. Cis and trans-fatty acids are not useful nutritional substances and if consumed regularly in large amounts can have negative effects on your cardiovascular system. I recommend that you use a spread such as tahini, avocado and houmos instead of margarine on your bread and crackers.

SALT — SODIUM CHLORIDE
Salt is a compound of two elements, sodium and chloride. Forty per cent of salt is sodium and 60% is chloride. Our nutritional requirement for sodium is only 250–350mg each day. If one level teaspoon of salt contains 2000mg of sodium, then it is easy to understand why many of us eat too much of it. Excess salt in the diet will increase your risk of high blood pressure, cardiovascular disease, fluid retention and osteoporosis.

Many menopausal women consume excess salt which is not surprising when you consider how much salt is added to processed and convenience foods or what standard additions to the dinner table are the salt and pepper shakers.

There are several things you should do in order to reduce your sodium intake. Read labels on processed foods and avoid products that contain salt or sodium in any form. Watch for hidden sodium in the form of flavour enhancers and preservatives like monosodium glutamate (MSG). MSG is usually listed as food additive number 621 on food labels. Occasionally, it is included in salt shakers at fast food outlets and adds a different flavour to chips and chicken. Artificial sweeteners can also contain high levels of sodium. Reducing your intake of processed and fast foods usually leads to a large reduction of dietary sodium levels. Stop adding salt to your cooking and put away the salt shaker. At first you will miss the salty taste. You may have strong cravings for salt for the first few months but they will pass and eventually your tastebuds will readjust and you will be able to taste the subtle flavours of foods again.

SUPPLEMENTS FOR A HEALTHY HEART AND BLOOD VESSELS

Vitamins A, C, E and betacarotene, known as the antioxidant nutrients reduce damage to the blood vessels caused by free radicals (see Page 101). Find a good quality antioxidant tablet containing all of these vitamins and take 2 tablets every day. A study conducted at Boston's Brigham and Women's Hospital and the Harvard School of Public Health showed that daily supplementation with vitamin E in doses of between 100–400iu, reduced the risk of heart attack by 25–50% in both sexes.

Garlic is the most popular food herb in the world today. It contains compounds such as sulphur amino acids, antioxidants, selenium and allicin which exert beneficial effects on the blood vessels and immune system. It acts as a natural body cleanser and antibiotic. Best of all it reduces unfavourable LDL cholesterol and reduces the tendency to form blood clots. You may eat it fresh or cooked in your meals or take odourless garlic capsules, 1–2 grams of garlic daily is a suitable dose.

Magnesium is a mineral vital for heart muscle relaxation and improves metabolic function and energy production in the heart muscle and blood vessel walls[15]. Many menopausal women suffer with an irregular or racing heart beat (palpitations) associated with hot flushes and this can be helped by taking magnesium.

Good dietary sources of magnesium are wheatgerm, nuts, legumes, whole grains, all dark green vegetables, dolomite and milk.

You can obtain magnesium chelate tablets and recommended doses are 400–800mg daily. Your doctor can check your magnesium level with a blood test.

MISCELLANEOUS SUPPLEMENTS

The herbs Ginkgo Biloba and Bilberry contain bioflavonoids that have a vitamin C like action and strengthen the tiny blood vessels (capillaries) in your cardiovascular system. They are available as tablets or capsules from your pharmacy or health food store. Take 2–6 capsules daily. The supplement Co-enzyme Q10 plays an important role in energy production in the heart, brain and body muscles.

FOODS FOR HEALTHY BONES

Generally speaking, for healthy bones women require 800–1000mg of calcium daily. During pregnancy, lactation and menopause, calcium needs increase to 1000–1500mg daily.

Check to see if your daily diet provides you with these amounts of calcium (see Table 13). If your diet on any one day falls short of this, or if you are not sure, take a good quality calcium tablet to give you 1000mg of calcium daily.

One of the best sources of calcium is milk and you will see from Table 13 that a cup of milk daily will give you a good start to meeting your daily requirements. When it comes to cows' milk, I recommend calcium-enriched milk such as Shape or Physical, which are low in fat and much higher in calcium than skim milk. If you are on a dairy-free diet you may choose soy milk and goats' or sheep milk products instead. You will see in the Calcium Table that some soy milks are calcium enriched while others are low in calcium and it is best to choose the former.

Our bones also contain the trace minerals zinc, silica, boron and manganese, as well as calcium. If your diet is not always perfect, I suggest you take a trace mineral tablet, such as Organic Mineral Formula, which contains all these trace minerals. Take 1 Organic Mineral Formula tablet daily along with your calcium tablet. Calcium and mineral tablets are best taken last thing at night, before retiring.

GOOD CALCIUM FOODS

FOOD	AVERAGE SERVE	MILLIGRAMS OF CALCIUM
Whole milk	250 ml (1 cup)	300
Shape milk	250 ml (1 cup)	408
Skim milk	250 ml (1 cup)	300
Physical/Hi-Lo/Lite White	250 ml (1 cup)	355
Goats' milk	250 ml (1 cup)	295
So Good Lite	250 ml (1 cup)	290
Creamy Original Vitasoy	250 ml (1 cup)	80
Soy Aussie Lite	250 ml (1 cup)	325
Powdered skim milk	1 tablespoon	130
Natural yoghurt/ low-fat natural yoghurt	200 g	240
Reduced-fat block cheese	30 g (3 cm cube)	258
Fetta cheese	30 g	129
Low-fat cottage cheese	30 g	35
Ricotta	30 g	100
Egg	60 g	35
Sardines	100 g	350
Salmon	100 g	190
Tuna (with bones)	100 g	290
Fish (fresh, cooked)	100 g	35
Almonds (unsalted)	30 g (25 nuts/average)	70
Brazil nuts (unsalted)	30 g (7-8 nuts)	55
Walnuts (unsalted)	30 g (25 nuts/average)	30
Pistachio nuts (unsalted)	30 g (23 nuts/average)	40
Whole sesame seeds	30 g (2½ tablespoons)	290
Sunflower seeds	30 g (2½ tablespoons)	30
Rhubarb	½ cup (cooked)	170
Orange	1	30
Rockmelon	½	30
Fresh fruit	each piece (average)	10–30
Broccoli	1 cup	50
Spinach	1 cup	100
Vegetables	1 cup (average)	10–50
Chick peas	½ cup	75
Baked beans	½ cup	60
Kidney beans	½ cup	60
Soy beans	½ cup	90
Bread (average all types)	1 slice	30
Cereal (average all types)	30 g	5–30
Tahini (sesame paste)	1 tablespoon	85
Houmos	1 tablespoon	15
Tofu	½ cup (130 g)	130

TABLE 13

CHAPTER 11

CAN I SLOW DOWN THE AGEING PROCESS?

As a doctor I find that a significant percentage of women are worried that the onset of menopause signals a sudden increase in their rate of ageing and that their looks will fade overnight. This will not occur if we learn how to reduce the factors that determine the ageing process.

The rate at which we age is determined by several factors. The ones you can't control are your genetic inheritance and the age at which you pass through the menopause.

The factors over which you *can* exert control are exercise, diet and lifestyle, exposure to the sun's ultra violet rays and your immune system.

1. Exercise

Exercise is vital for women in midlife as, after the menopause, the metabolic rate decreases causing a tendency to easy weight gain and in 50% of post-menopausal women there is an increase in body weight of five kilograms and in many cases much more. Ideally, at least 20 to 30 minutes of aerobic exercise should be done daily to stimulate the heart, circulation of blood and respiration. This can consist of doing aerobic exercise to music at a gym or in your own home, swimming, aqua aerobics or jogging. For those who have not done any aerobic exercise before, the process should be started gradually, starting with five minutes a day and increasing during a four-week period to thirty minutes daily. For those women with cardiovascular risk factors such as obesity, smoking, high cholesterol, diabetes, high blood pressure or a poor family history of heart disease, a full fitness check-up including a cardiac stress test should be done by a cardiologist before aerobic exercise is undertaken. For those with arthritic joints and backache, aerobics, jogging and strenuous weight-bearing exercise may aggravate pain and damage. For those people, modified yoga, tai chi or swimming and walking are excellent as they stretch the joints gradually and keep the muscles in tone.

Many menopausal women find that aerobic exercise can be awkward because of stress incontinence. This means that when the intra-abdominal pressure is increased by exercise, straining, coughing, etc., urine is passed uncontrollably soiling the underclothes. This happens because a deficiency of the female hormones can cause the pelvic floor muscles to weaken and sag so that the bladder is insufficiently supported.

Exercises to strengthen the pelvic floor muscles can overcome stress incontinence in 40–50% of cases. See Page 114 to learn pelvic floor exercises.

2. The Anti-Ageing Diet

A woman in midlife need not be fanatical about diet as obsessions can cause an early death through stress or boredom. There are some basic principles that should be followed for profound and far-reaching benefits to your physical and mental wellbeing. These principles are:

i) Learn to love RAW vegetables and fruits. Ideally around 50% of the dietary intake should consist of raw foods. Raw foods are living foods and by virtue of this they will stimulate the metabolism and aid the elimination of toxic waste materials from the body. Raw foods contain beneficial molecules such as antioxidants and Indoles, which have anti-cancer properties and are excellent in overcoming obesity, arthritis and high blood pressure. Ideally, women in midlife should buy themselves a juice extracting machine with which to make raw vegetable and fruit juices on a daily basis. Juices not only supply essential minerals and vitamins but also contain easily assimilated organic compounds such as vegetable amino acids that function similarly to some of the body secretions and hormones. Raw fruit and vegetable juices are distinct and incomparable in the rejuvenation and regeneration of the human organism. No other source supplies as much vitamin C as fruits and vegetables, and this vitamin is entirely destroyed when the juices are subjected to heat.

Generally, half a litre of juice daily is the least that will show worthwhile results. If you can manage more, all the better, and one litre may be needed to stimulate a quicker process of detoxification and rejuvenation.

Recommended juice combinations are:

A. Several of the following — apple, grapefruit, orange, strawberry, pear, pineapple, peach.

B. Several of the following — carrot, celery, tomatoe, parsley, cucumber, cabbage, spinach, beetroot, radish, dandelion, lettuce, turnip leaf juice, watercress.

C. For health cocktails add a dash of lemon, strawberry and honey.

ii) Avoid processed chemical and frozen foods and buy foods in their natural state as they contain more fibre and less calories and fat. Choose unprocessed grains, cereals, seeds, nuts, legumes and wholegrain bread instead of products made with white flour, white sugar, colourings, salt, commercial sauces and processed fats.

iii) Reduce fats, not just cholesterol, but all saturated fats. This means you will need to avoid fatty meats such as lamb, pork and chicken with the skin, processed meats, preserved meats, fried foods, coconut, some processed margarines and full-fat dairy products. You should especially avoid fats that have turned rancid, as they generate the production of free radicals, which will increase inflammation and cancer formation.

Substitute saturated fats with polyunsaturated fats by eating foods such as grilled fish, seeds, grains, legumes, almonds, vegetables and cold-pressed vegetable and seed oils.

iv) Drink 8–12 glasses of water daily. The best type of water is that passed through a water purifier which can be attached easily to your kitchen tap. Water will dilute the blood thereby reducing cholesterol and acidity and improving a sluggish circulation.

3. The Immune System

Your immune system is the defence and surveillance system that protects your cells against infections, toxins, free radicals and non-specific damage. The immune system is very complex and consists of the lymphatic system, liver, spleen, bone marrow and thymus gland. The thymus gland situated in the lower part of the neck, and behind the breast plate or sternum is the master gland of the immune system and orchestrates the other parts.

Unfortunately, the valuable thymus gland shrinks with age which leads to a general reduction in the efficiency of the immune system. As our ageing immune system weakens, we become more susceptible to degeneration and inflammation of our cells, infections, cancer and more rapid ageing. All of these things may add up eventually to shorten our life span.

Thus, you can comprehend the huge importance of a healthy immune system in the quest for youthfulness and a longer life span. The immune system acts to reduce damage and ageing of the most vulnerable parts of our cells, such as the nucleus and intra-cellular metabolic structures.

FREE RADICALS

To understand the process of ageing it is essential that you know about 'free radicals'. These sound like political terrorists and indeed they are dangerous, unstable electronic particles that terrorise our cells. They rush around the body damaging cell walls, genetic material, blood vessel walls, joints and intra-cellular components. When free radicals are produced in your skin, they damage collagen fibres, causing cross-linkage and degeneration of collagen resulting in wrinkling, thinning and ageing of the skin. These horrible evil free radicals cause an atomic bomb-type chain reaction in our precious cells, which keeps on generating more and more free radicals. Obviously, we all hate free radicals as they damage our cells, leading to more rapid ageing, and all of us would like to reduce their production in our bodies.

Although free radicals are inevitable to some degree, as they are formed when we are exposed to polluted air, cigarette smoke, rancid dietary fats, some highly processed chemical foods, fluorescent lights, video display units, viruses and alcohol, there is still a great deal we can do to protect our cells against their destructive effects.

ANTIOXIDANTS
Vitamin E

One of the greatest methods existing to protect our tender tissues from free radical damage is to take vitamin E. Vitamin E has been recognised for many years for its anti-ageing effect, long before scientists understood the significance and existence of free radicals.

One word of caution, however, is that only the natural forms of vitamin E are useful and, unfortunately, thousands of women are erroneously taking the synthetic form of vitamin E, which is of negligible use. The natural forms of vitamin E are called D-tocopherols. These D-tocopherols are a mixture of alpha, beta, gamma, delta, eta, epsilon and zeta and they all play a valuable role in scavenging and neutralising free radicals. Studies seem to indicate that doses between 500 and 1,000 international units a day can help to slow down the ageing process. You can also find vitamin E in fresh wheat germ, nuts, eggs and cold pressed oils such as soyabean, olive, sunflower, sesame and safflower.

According to an American cancer specialist, Dr Jeffrey Blumberg from Tufts University, Boston, the incidence of cancer could be halved by increasing antioxidants through dietary changes and nutritional supplements. Vitamin E can inhibit cancer development in the skin, breast and colon. Dr Blumberg has found compelling evidence that we can add years to a healthy life by taking sufficient antioxidants. To achieve this he recommends taking supplements or eating 5–9 servings of fresh fruit and vegetables each day.

Beta-Carotene

Another free radical protector is the nutritional substance called Beta-Carotene which is found in high concentration in certain vegetables such as carrots, silverbeet leaf and pumpkin and that is one of the reasons why raw vegetable juices are so wonderfully good for age-conscious folks. If you take too much Beta Carotene your skin may turn a slightly yellow or bronze colour as the carotene is a yellow pigment. This is harmless and is not equivalent to vitamin A overdosage and if it happens, simply reduce your intake of Beta Carotene until the bronze colour fades. It is possible to take Beta Carotene in supplement form and tablets of 6mg can safely be taken in a dose of 1 to 3 tablets daily. Beta Carotene is converted in the liver into vitamin A and this is beneficial as vitamin A is in itself a powerful free radical scavenger and so a useful anti-ageing substance. It is especially important for the strength and metabolism of the skin and mucous membranes which are particularly vulnerable to drying and infection in menopausal women. Doses of 5,000 to 10,000 international units daily are helpful in those with a normal liver function, but if you suffer with any medical disorders, check with your doctor first before taking vitamin A.

Vitamin C

The miracle anti-ageing and rejuvenating properties of vitamin C, are to the water soluble parts of your body what vitamin E is to the fatty parts. Vitamin C is a powerful antioxidant and free radical scavenger and is extremely important in maintaining the integrity and elasticity of collagen in your skin and bones. Vitamin C will reduce ageing of your skin and bones. The best sources of vitamin C are fresh fruits and vegetables but as an insurance policy, I recommend that all women take a supplement of the calcium ascorbate powder form of vitamin C in a dosage of 1000mg twice daily, which is easily dissolved in raw fruit and vegetable juices. According to Dr. Judie Walton, a gerentologist at the Ageing Research Institute at Concord Hospital, vitamins E and C prolong life in experimental animals and she expects the same is true for humans. Dr. Walton says that this is logical as, if antioxidant vitamins protect our specialised cells, these cells will not need to be replenished so often from our cell banks which will last longer and life span should increase accordingly. The non-acidic form of vitamin C ascorbate is better for people who find the ascorbic acid form too acidic. Calcium ascorbate is the best vitamin C for menopausal women as it also provides some calcium. Some people become hypersensitive or allergic to vitamin C supplements, even Ester C which is normally well tolerated. If so, eat foods high in vitamin C such as fresh raw fruits and vegetables.

ESSENTIAL FATTY ACIDS

These are unsaturated fats that are essential to eat for health and vitality. They are essential for two reasons:

1. Our bodies are unable to manufacture them.
2. Our cells cannot function normally without them.

If a patient of mine asks me what is the most important supplement for health and beauty, I would respond "essential fatty acids". This is because the membranes that surround and protect each cell in our body are made of essential fatty acids (EFAs).

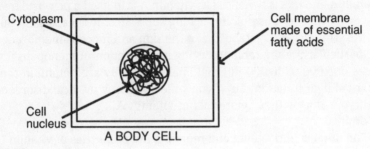

Cytoplasm

Cell membrane made of essential fatty acids

Cell nucleus

A BODY CELL

DIAGRAM 10

The physical integrity and energy production of our cells depends upon adequate amounts of EFAs in the diet.

If our cell membranes break down or weaken, they may no longer be able to prevent dangerous particles (e.g. toxic chemicals, infective organisms, viruses and free radicals) from passing through them. If such dangerous particles manage to pass through the weakened cell membrane, they enter the inner sanctum of the cell where they may inflict severe damage. Such damage may be irreparable and result in physical, chemical and electrical impairment of the cell. If widespread this may result in chronic inflammation and degeneration and increase the rate of ageing of our cells. If the cell nucleus containing the genetic control centre of the cell is severely damaged the cell may be transformed into a cancer cell.

So you can understand why it is vital to have strong, healthy membranes around your cells to protect the inner sanctum of these cells. This is one of the most important strategies for slowing down the ageing process and enabling us to look, feel and function younger for longer.

Essential fatty acids are the most important nutrients to build and maintain strong and efficient cell membranes.

The antioxidants — vitamins A, C, E, beta carotene and selenium—also help our cell membranes to keep out these nasty invaders like free radicals and viruses.

If we thought of an analogy, a good one would be to see a body cell as a castle. The cell membrane is the moat and brick wall around the castle, while the antioxidants are the army of men, shooting bullets to weaken and inactivate the castle's invaders.

Where do we obtain EFAs? They can be found in certain foods (such as fish, grains, beans and seed oils), breast milk and nutritional supplements.

SOURCES AND FUNCTIONS OF ESSENTIAL FATTY ACIDS

FOODS	ESSENTIAL FATTY ACIDS	PROSTAGLANDIN FAMILY	EFFECT IN BODY
SOURCES OF OMEGA 6 EFAs Sesame, sunflower seeds and oil, (cold-pressed), blackcurrant seeds and their oil, evening primrose oil, borage oil, spirulina, soya beans, lecithin.	Linoleic acid, gamma linolenic acid.	Prostaglandin 1 is the first body messenger (desirable).	Reduces pain and inflammation. Improves skin. Increases energy and vitality.
SOURCES OF OMEGA 3 EFAs Linseed oil, blackcurrant seeds and their oils, cod liver oil, mackeral and fresh fish from cold deep oceans, sardines, tuna, salmon (must not be fried), fish oil capsules.	Alpha linolenic acid, eicosapentaenoic acid (EPA).	Prostaglandin 3 (desirable).	Reduces pain and inflammation. Helps circulation.
SOURCES OF SATURATED FATS Saturated fats in animal meats, full-cream dairy products, preserved meats, fried foods, processed and take away meals, coconut palm oil.	Arachidonic acid.	Prostaglandin 2 (undesirable).	Excess amounts of these foods may increase pain and inflammation and can result in sticky platelets and poor circulation.

.TABLE 14

There are two types or families of beneficial EFAs, namely omega 6 and omega 3. Omega 6 EFAs are linoleic and gamma linolenic acid.

Omega 3 EFAs are alpha linolenic and eicosapentaenoic acids. Table 14 shows you which foods and supplements provide you with omega 6 and omega 3 EFAs respectively.

EFAs not only strengthen your cell membranes, they also help to balance the vitally important hormone-like chemicals called Prostaglandins. There are three families of Prostaglandins — Prostaglandin 1 (PG1), Prostaglandin 2(PG2), and Prostaglandin 3(PG3). Let's call them PG1, PG2 and PG3.

The PG1 and PG3 families are beneficial to the body because they reduce inflammation and regulate the function of many hormonal glands and also the brain's chemistry. Omega 6 EFAs produce PG1 and Omega 3 EFAs produce PG3 (see Table 14). This is desirable and promotes a healthy immune system. In particular, PG1 acts as the first messenger in the body and increases production and release of many different hormones and brain chemicals (neurotransmitters). Thus, omega 6 EFAs, by making PG1, keep your hormonal glands and brain cells "switched on".

PG1 increases the production and release of hormones such as thyroid hormone, cortisone, growth hormone and sex hormones. PG1 also increases the production and release of brain chemicals called neurotransmitters. Because of this, women with mental fatigue, emotional imbalance, chronic fatigue syndrome and adrenal gland exhaustion should take omega 6 EFAs to boost their PG1 levels. The best ways of increasing your intake of EFAs is to take supplements of evening primrose oil, linseed (flaxseed) oil, blackcurrant seed oil and fish oil—see Table 14 for a comprehensive list. Also include fresh and canned fish, seeds, vegetables and cold pressed seed oils regularly in the diet.

The recommended dose of evening primrose oil is 2–4 grams daily.

Increasing your intake of EFAs will help you in many ways. It will:

1. Improve the appearance and health of your skin, hair and nails.
2. Increase mental and physical energy.
3. Boost your immune system.
4. Reduce inflammation and aches and pains.
5. Improve your circulation and reduce cardiovascular disease.
6. Reduce cellular damage and thereby slow down the rate of ageing and reduce your risk of cancer.
7. Reduce breast pain and tenderness.
8. Improve gynaecological health by reducing period pain, ovarian cysts and pelvic inflammation.

As we age, our bodies become less efficient at manufacturing PG1 and PG3 and this is partly why we slow down and suffer increasing aches and pains with advancing years. Also, as we age, and especially if our diet is high in saturated fats (see Table 14), we produce increasing amounts of the undesirable PG2 family of hormone-like chemicals. PG2 acts in the body to increase inflammation and pain. Many menopausal and post-menopausal women complain of a variety of painful syndromes from headaches, arthritis and rheumatics to back ache. This is largely due to an imbalance in their prostaglandins — too much PG2 and not enough PG1 and PG3. In such cases, doctors may prescribe anti-inflammatory drugs known as anti-prostaglandin drugs to suppress the body's production of PG2. These drugs work quickly and efficiently to relieve pain and inflammation, but if taken for many months may cause unpleasant side effects.

If my patients complain of pain and inflammation in their muscles, bones and joints, I prefer to teach them how to reduce these problems with nutritional medicine, rather than rely on anti-inflammatory drugs alone. This is not hard to do. You should simply:

1. Reduce saturated fats in your diet.
2. Increase omega 3 + omega 6 essential fatty acids (EFAs) in the diet (see Table 14).
3. Take antioxidants regularly.
4. Drink 1–2 litres of water daily and raw vegetable juices.

The essential fatty acid story sounds too good to be true. I have been recommending EFAs to thousands of women with poor health and I can assure you that it is worthwhile to increase the EFAs in your diet. As we age, we need to "oil but not grease" to slow down the ageing process.

If you would like to know more about research into EFAs you could refer to: Dr Stephen Wright MD, Royal Free Hospital, School of Medicine in London. The books *Heal Cancer* by Dr Ruth Cilento MD, published by Hill of Content, Australia, and *Fats and Oils* by Udo Erasmus BSc, published by Alive Books in Canada.

ANTI AGEING HORMONES
Growth Hormone
A powerful hormone involved in the ageing process is Growth Hormone which is produced by the pituitary gland. During normal ageing, growth hormone production decreases from about age 20 to very low levels in some

people by age 60. This is usually accompanied by reductions in muscle mass, metabolic rate, muscle strength, exercise performance and an increase in cholesterol. Thus, normal ageing is growth hormone-related. A deficiency of growth hormone causes fatigue, increased body fat especially around the stomach, slight reduction in muscle mass, cold hands and feet, feeling cold and sometimes sexual dysfunction. Growth hormone deficiency affects men and women in equal numbers.

There is no question that people with an abnormal lack of growth hormone should receive treatment, and recently American scientists have found that a group of healthy men aged between 61 and 81 emerged with bodies almost 20 years younger after receiving injections of growth hormone. Injections of growth hormone have been shown to increase lean body tissue, muscle mass and exercise performance while reducing body fat and cholesterol.

You will be happy to know that regular exercise seems to promote the production of your own growth hormone from the pituitary gland. Simply by exercising regularly you are slowing down the ageing process by increasing your own supplies of precious growth hormone in a natural way.

The Thymus Gland

Going back to the pivotal role of the master thymus gland, exciting new research in Europe and the USA shows that injections of extracts from the thymus gland may increase the resistance of the immune system in animals and when these injections have been used in human beings they have often produced a feeling of rejuvenation in the recipients. Further research could very well reveal that taking extracts of thymus will slow down ageing of the immune system.

The Thyroid Gland

It is not uncommon for the thyroid gland to become slightly underactive at the time of the menopause and indeed women are far more prone to thyroid disease than men. The thyroid gland controls the metabolic rate and if it becomes underactive, the metabolic rate will reduce causing easy weight gain, difficulty in losing weight, dry thickened skin, dry thinning hair, constipation, sensitivity to cold and mental slowness. Your thyroid gland can be checked by a simple blood test. If it is found to be underactive you will be prescribed thyroid hormone which will re-establish the metabolic rate and cause a return to normal body weight and mental activity. If your metabolism is a little sluggish and you seem to have trouble burning up the calories, and yet your blood test shows that your thyroid gland is functioning within normal limits, you may be able to stimulate your metabolism by taking spirulina (a nutritional supplement) and dried macrobiotic seaweed preparations. These contain the essential mineral iodine along with other essential minerals to generally stimulate the metabolism.

CHAPTER 12

SEX AND MENOPAUSE

My patient Julie had had a hysterectomy for fibroids two years ago at the age of forty-seven and came to see me about her sex life which was in total disarray. Julie related that for twelve months she had not felt any sexual urges and that when she had sex it was merely to please her husband, who by all accounts was as virile as ever. During sex Julie found that she experienced a burning pain and tightness in her vagina and this would cause her to feel anxious and sweat profusely. Doctors use the term dyspareunia to describe painful sexual intercourse and Julie certainly fitted into this category. She also complained that stimulation of her clitoris was no longer pleasurable and indeed she had noticed that her clitoris was shrinking and felt tender and fragile.

"I'm definitely not the sexpot I used to be," Julie said and she felt that her husband was taking her lack of response personally, and was beginning to doubt his ability to be a passionate lover.

Examination of Julie's vagina showed it to be affected by lack of sex hormones—it was pale in colour and its mucous membranes were thin, dry and fragile. Her clitoris was very small, inflamed and tender. Thankfully, her ovaries felt normal and she had no sign of prolapse of the vagina. A blood test revealed that Julie's menopause had started because her levels of oestrogen and testosterone were very low.

Julie decided that she wanted to try HRT to bring her hormonal levels back into the normal range. I reassured her that HRT would reverse the ageing changes that had occurred in the sexual areas of her anatomy.

I gave Julie an injection of a mixture of natural oestrogen and testosterone called Primodian which acts like a "mini-implant" in that it restores the levels of the sex hormones, oestrogen and testosterone, in the body in the same way that a hormone implant does but for a shorter period of time.

Four weeks later Julie returned, saying, as I knew she would, that she had rediscovered her former sexual enthusiasm and was now able to enjoy sex, lubricate after stimulation and have satisfying orgasms. Her dyspareunia had vanished and she was also pleased that the oestrogen in the injection had made her shrinking breasts rounder and fuller.

Julie had enjoyed her mental and physical response to HRT and wanted to maintain the effect of the injection. I explained to her that the injection's effect would only last 6–8 weeks and that to continue feeling the way she felt now, the most effective strategy would be to insert an implant of 100mg of oestrogen and 100mg of testosterone into the fat of her buttocks. Such an implant would last for approximately twelve months, and she could then have another implant. This idea appealed to Julie as she could not be bothered with tablets or patches in her busy lifestyle which involved a lot of travel. Before inserting the implant, I warned Julie that the testosterone implant may cause a slight increase in facial pimples and hair, however for Julie this was a small price to pay. If you do not feel this way yourself, an implant of oestrogen alone can be used, which will help greatly with your sex life, but to a lesser degree than if you received both oestrogen and testosterone in your implant. Testosterone has the effects of increasing your libido (sex drive) and may cause slight enlargement of the clitoris. Some women choose to take testosterone initially in their long term programme of HRT, others choose to use it intermittently, say once every few years, while many women feel it is not for them at all. Your sexual needs may change as you age and your HRT can be modified to blend in with this.

FACTORS THAT REDUCE LIBIDO AT MENOPAUSE

1. Lack Of Sex Hormones

Deficiencies of oestrogen and testosterone often reduce sexual desire and produce shrinkage and dryness of the vagina and vaginal lips (see Diagram 12).

2. Poor General Health And Medical Problems

If you suffer with chronic fatigue, recurrent painful conditions or feel generally unwell, you will probably have a reduced interest in sexual activity as a result. To improve your general health, Chapters 10 and 11 will provide you with valuable information.

Women who smoke heavily often notice a big reduction in their sexual response as they age. This is because the phases of sexual excitement, lubrication and orgasm, are due to the congestion and swelling with blood of the erotic tissues in the clitoris, vulva and vagina. Smoking damages the small blood vessels all over the body, including in the vaginal areas and means that they are less able to swell up with blood in response to sexual stimulation. Thus, your sexual response can be impaired by heavy smoking.

3. Prescription Medications

A wide range of drugs may affect sexual function causing loss of libido, arousal difficulty and orgasmic dysfunction. The most common drugs to cause these problems are appetite suppressants, some muscle relaxants, some drugs for epilepsy, some drugs to prevent headaches, some drugs to treat high blood pressure, some sedatives and anti-depressant drugs, some anti-ulcer drugs and anti-male hormones. Make sure you check with your doctor before your begin taking a new medication as you may be upset if your sexual ability and desire become lessened by the medication. There is often a suitable alternative drug which will not do this as new derivatives of older drugs which have less side effects and no adverse effects on libido are becoming available regularly.

4. Vaginal Problems

Menopausal women may have two vaginal reasons why their sex life has deteriorated — namely, prolapse and/or dryness of the mucous membrane lining.

Prolapse

The term prolapse means a loosening and falling down of tissues or organs due to stretching and the force of gravity with advancing years. Common areas to prolapse are the uterus and front and back walls of the vagina (see Diagram 11). If the front wall of the vagina prolapses, the bladder often prolapses down into it, forming a swelling that can be seen when you cough. This combined bladder and vaginal prolapse is called a cystocele. Women with a cystocele often have problems with stress incontinence—meaning when they cough, strain or run, they pass urine involuntarily. If the back wall of the vagina prolapses, the lower bowel (rectum) often prolapses down into it, forming a swelling that may fill with faeces especially if you are constipated. This swelling is called a rectocele (see Diagram 11).

If the uterus prolapses down into the vagina, a more solid swelling can be felt or seen and in severe cases, the cervix protrudes outside of the vaginal opening. Women with a uterine prolapse have usually had several children or experienced difficult and prolonged labour.

With all these types of prolapse, it is easy to understand why sexual intercourse may be uncomfortable and perhaps a little embarrassing. Also, with prolapse, the vaginal and pelvic floor muscles are stretched to such a degree that both the woman and her partner find the vagina is too big for either to feel very much during intercourse. In moderate to severe cases of prolapse a surgical vaginal repair is necessary and can be done completely through incisions in the vagina. A vaginal repair will eliminate a cystocele or rectocele, reduce or cure stress incontinence and make your vagina a normal snug size so that sexual intercourse once again becomes enjoyable.

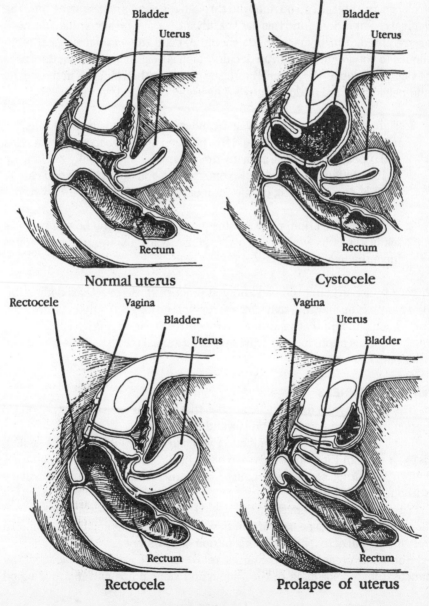

Normal uterus

Cystocele

Rectocele

Prolapse of uterus

DIAGRAM 11

If your uterus has prolapsed down into the vagina, you will probably have a dull, dragging discomfort in your pelvic and vaginal areas. You have the choice of removing the uterus (hysterectomy) or having the uterine ligaments repaired so that the uterus is no longer prolapsed. In most cases of uterine prolapse, the uterus can be removed through the vagina, at the same time the vaginal repair is done, and this has the advantage that no abdominal incisions are required. Your gynaecologist should explain the various surgical techniques to you in full before you decide which is best for you. In milder cases of vaginal prolapse, the "Kegel Exercises" to strengthen muscles in the vagina and pelvic floor are often effective. These can be done two ways:

1. Tighten and squeeze your vagina and rectum by drawing their muscles inwards and upwards and hold this position for 5–10 seconds, then relax and repeat the exercise as many times as possible, gradually working up to 100–200 times each day. No one can see you doing it and you can do it while driving, sitting on the train or watching TV etc.

2. While passing urine, practise starting and stopping the flow of urine as many times as you can. This exercise will help women with stress incontinence.

If your prolapse is not too bad and you practise these exercises daily, after 3–4 months you may find that surgical repair is no longer needed. As an added bonus you will find that your muscular control of the vagina and pelvic floor during sex has improved, thus giving greater sexual pleasure to both you and your partner.

VAGINAL DRYNESS

There are several different strategies that you can use singly or in combination to overcome vaginal dryness and fragility.

For a temporary lubrication action you can use bland jellies such as K-Y Jelly or vitamin E cream which also has a healing effect. These can be used before or during sexual intercourse and are available at your pharmacy without a prescription.

To restore and strengthen the vagina and vulva, you will need to use hormonal creams, especially if you have had an early menopause or want to resume sexual activity after a long period of abstinence.

Hormonal creams and pessaries rejuvenate, thicken and moisten the mucosal folds and lining of the vagina and vaginal lips and improve blood circulation to the clitoral area, thus restoring capacity for natural lubrication and orgasm. If you feel that your vagina has shrunk and is too small for the penis of your partner, this can be overcome by regularly massaging the inside and opening of the vaginal walls using an oestrogen cream. Place some oestrogen cream on your fingers and rub it into the vaginal walls, gently stretching apart the walls and exert gentle pressure backwards at the opening of the vagina. This can be done gradually more and more each day and there is no need to stretch excessively and cause any discomfort. Ten minutes daily of this gentle massage and stretching is sufficient and it is most comfortable to do it lying down. Oestrogen creams and pessaries require a prescription as they contain hormones and various suitable brands are Dienoestrol, Premarin, Ovestin and Kolpon. In some women, especially if the clitoris has become very small, the addition of testosterone to the vaginal oestrogen cream can be much

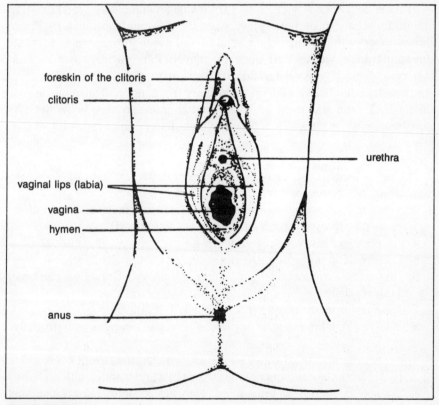

DIAGRAM 12

more effective in restoring the sexual response of the vagina, vaginal lips and clitoris.

The clitoris is normally the size of a large pea—see Diagram 12 to see it's relative size.

You can ask your doctor to write you a prescription for a vaginal cream containing both oestrogen and testosterone as follows:

The Cream = 40% oestrogen cream, 20% testosterone cream made from 3 ampoules of Primoteston Depot injections, 20% vaseline, 20% sorbolene and glycerine.

You may massage your vagina, vulva and clitoris with this cream every night for 3–4 weeks, after which time you will only need to use the cream twice a week.

Some of my patients have told me that their hormonal creams or pessaries act like an aphrodisiac and make them feel more sexy!

In some menopausal women, recurrent vaginal and bladder inflammation and/or infections make them feel very tender, itchy and most unsexy. These things occur partly because the sexual tissues are more vulnerable to infections and trauma without hormones and your HRT and vaginal creams should take care of this. If your vagina and vulva remain tender and inflamed and you continue to suffer bladder infections, urinary frequency and burning, despite taking HRT, you will need to boost your immune system with diet and nutritional supplements. To boost your immune system, I recommend that you:

1. Drink 2 litres of purified or bottled water daily.
2. Drink 2–3 glasses of raw vegetable juices daily.
3. Avoid refined sugar, foods containing refined sugar, alcohol, coffee, cigarettes and yeast products (eat yeast free bread).
4. Eat plenty of raw vegetables and fruit.
5. Take evening primrose oil, 3 grams daily.
6. Take an antioxidant tablet containing vitamin A, C, E and Beta carotene, 2 tablets daily.
7. Take garlic or odourless garlic capsules, 1–2 grams daily.
8. Take acidophilus capsules or powder or eat acidophilus yoghurt daily.

These simple and safe strategies are extremely effective in overcoming recurrent infections or inflammation in the vagina and bladder, although they may take several months to bring relief. They are certainly safer than taking frequent courses of antibiotic drugs which in the long term only weaken your own immune system. Please see your doctor if symptoms persist.

TESTS FOR WOMEN WITH A POOR SEX DRIVE

If you are worried by a lack of sex drive, ask your doctor to do a blood test to measure various hormones that are important determinants of libido and sexual wellbeing. It does not matter if you are already taking HRT, as some women on HRT still find that their sex life is poor. This could mean that your HRT needs adjusting.

The Blood Test Should Measure:

1. Follicle Stimulating Hormone (FSH)

If this is very high, say above 50mu/L, then you may benefit from a larger dose of oestrogen in your HRT. See Page 20 to refresh your memory of FSH.

2. Oestradiol

This is the biochemical name for oestrogen and if your level is less than 200pmol/L, you may benefit from a larger dose or different form of oestrogen. Some women on oestrogen tablets have a very active liver which breaks down the oestrogen as soon as it is absorbed from the intestine and passes through the liver. In other words, the liver may weaken the effect of the oestrogen before it has a chance to work on your mind and sexual organs. Such women may find that they need increasing doses of oestrogen tablets to feel normal and yet their blood oestrogen levels remain low. Of course, one cannot go on increasing the dose of oestrogen tablets indefinitely as side effects such as nausea, fluid retention and breast swelling may result.

If your liver is too active and your oestrogen tablets are no longer relieving your symptoms, I suggest your ask your doctor about forms of oestrogen that bypass the liver—namely, patches, injections or implants.

Some women find that by inserting their oestrogen tablets high into the vagina, instead of taking them by mouth, they get a better result because the oestrogen tablets are absorbed directly into the bloodstream from the vagina and thus bypass the liver.

For these reasons, some women find that their libido and sexual response improves after transfering to a form of oestrogen replacement therapy that is not taken by mouth.

3. Sex Hormone Binding Globulin (SHBG)

This is a protein produced by the liver and its function is to bind sex hormones such as oestrogen, progesterone and testosterone and carry them around in the circulation. In much the same way as a car transports you along a freeway, SHBG transports your sex hormones along your blood vessels. Sex hormone binding globulin binds your sex hormones and in this bound state they are not active in your body. Thus, if you have too much sex hormone binding globulin, the majority of your sex hormones will be bound and inactive. Chances are that as a result you will feel not only sexless but tired and grumpy.

What we like to see is that your SHBG falls somewhere in the middle of the normal range which is 30–90nmol/L. In other words, it is not desirable to have too little or too much SHBG.

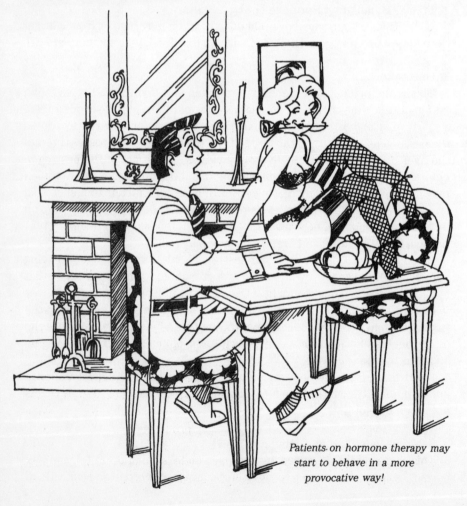

Patients on hormone therapy may start to behave in a more provocative way!

I see many women complaining of lost sexuality and in many of these cases I find that their blood test reveals very high levels of SHBG. Why is this? Once again, you can blame the liver and it is the oral forms of oestrogen that most stimulate the liver to produce increased amounts of SHBG. If your SHBG is high (90 or more) you may find that your sex life and general energy level improves by transferring to a non-oral form of oestrogen e.g. patches, implants, injections or take your oestrogen tablet via your vagina. By bypassing the liver in this way, the liver will be less stimulated into making SHBG and your levels of SHBG should start to fall.

If you have high levels of SHBG you may need a small dose of testosterone as SHBG also binds the hormone testosterone, thus inactivating it. Testosterone is best given in the form of implants or injections and can really bring the zing back into a tired sex life.

4. Male Hormones

These are also known as androgens. Women require some male hormones in their bodies (albeit much less than men) to give them a healthy sex drive and general mental and physical wellbeing.

We can measure the levels of these male hormones and the tests that are useful are the measurement of total testosterone, free testosterone and free androgens. The free male hormones are the ones not bound by SHBG and are thus the active male hormones in your body. If your doctor finds that your free testosterone and free androgens are very low this could very well explain your loss of sex drive and fatigue. If so, these problems are easily overcome by receiving some testosterone in the form of injections or implants.

Your State Of Mind

Some women find that the menopause is a time of sexual liberation and that their sex life becomes better than ever. This may be because they no longer have the worry of pregnancy and contraception and also because they have more time, space and privacy to have a relaxed sex life. By the age of 40, most women have become aware of their sexual needs and preferences and feel comfortable about telling their partner how to please them. This is a wonderful thing and if you are not able to fully express your sexual identity to your partner, it is very important that you try to improve communication or seek counselling.

Whether you are married, have an older or younger lover, the menopause and the years surrounding it can bring you great sexual satisfaction.

CHAPTER 13

THE MALE MENOPAUSE—FACT OR FICTION

This chapter is designed for you and your partner if he has a midlife crisis.

The word "menopause" literally means the cessation of menstrual bleeding. In females it signifies that the biological clock has stopped and infertility sets in accompanied by dramatic hormonal changes. So, the word "menopause" cannot apply to men. Yet, even though they seem to be on easy street compared to women, it is indeed a fact that men also are vulnerable to fundamental emotional, mental and physical changes at about 50 years of age and beyond when Hormone Replacement Therapy (HRT) may be of help to men as well as women.

The first semblance of Hormone Replacement Therapy (HRT) was used on a man in 1889, when a famous neurophysiologist Charles-Edouard Brown-Sequard, gave himself an extract of animal testicles. In his own words this produced "a return of vigour, youthful appetites and desires" due to the male hormone testosterone contained in the animal testicles.

HORMONAL CHANGES IN MEN

Testosterone production from the testicles is at its peak during the 20s and 30s and thereafter a slow decline occurs which becomes more pertinent after the age of 50. Despite this, there is a large variation between individual males so that some men at 50 may produce such low levels of testosterone that they no longer feel any inclination to have a sex life, whereas others at 80 have high testosterone levels and are still sexually vigorous. As you are reading this you are probably wondering how you (if you are male) or your partner can be one of the lucky ones and nurture those testicles all the way along throughout life. The ability to produce testosterone is partly genetic so that in many cases it's "like father, like son". We also know that lifestyle plays a role and men who smoke and/or drink alcohol excessively will have lower levels of testosterone in their blood.

As a man ages, not only does the production of testosterone diminish but so does the ability of his tissues and cells to respond to testosterone. It is a simple matter for a man to see if his testosterone production is down by asking for a blood test.

A deficiency of testosterone would be obvious if the blood level was below 8nmol/L, the normal range of testosterone for men in the blood being 11–37nmol/L. This would be further corroborated by high blood levels of the pituitary hormone called Luteinising Hormone (LH) which is indicative that the pituitary gland is trying to stimulate the sluggish testicles. This blood test could be repeated on three separate occasions, at eight-weekly intervals to demonstrate any trends before deciding if male HRT is needed.

THE SYMPTOMS OF TESTOSTERONE DEFICIENCY

Testosterone deficiency shows up in:

1. Reduced libido, fatigue and behaviourial changes
2. Shrinkage (atrophy) of the muscles, testicles and penis and softening of the testicles
3. Reduce rate of growth of facial and body hair
4. Reduction in virility and ability to achieve orgasm. In severe cases, impotence

A male who has previously had high levels of testosterone may find that the decreasing testosterone levels that can begin to occur after the age of 50 produce subtle mental and physical changes even though his blood test reveals that his testosterone levels are still within the normal physiological range of 11–37 nmol/L. This is because his testosterone levels are much lower than they used to be and he is sensitive to the decreasing levels.

Subtle changes of decreasing testosterone production may range from depression, loss of confidence, loss of drive and aggression and loss of competitiveness in all spheres. The warrior man finds himself becoming a bit of a mouse. If such a male takes himself along to the doctor he may be told that all this is symptomatic of the psychological male midlife crisis, especially after a full physical checkup fails to reveal any medical problems. He may be told that this crisis is due to a plateau in his career, looming retirement, unrealised ambitions, getting older, overdoing it, or stress.

He may be offered a course of anti-depressants, sedatives or tranquillisers and referred for counselling to assuage his growing self-doubts. Men are more reluctant than women to accept a course of such therapy preferring to numb their anxieties at the bar with their mates. Unfortunately, alcohol ingestion, if it becomes regular or excessive, often further reduces the production of testosterone leading to an aggravation of the mental and physical imbalance.

It is vital to check the possibility of a hormonal contribution and, if this is suspected, a short trial of HRT with testosterone can be tried.

The word "androgen" is the medical term for "male hormone".

Androgens may be given on a regular basis in tablet (oral) form. Some common brands are Testomet (methyltestosterone) or the relative new Andriol (testosterone undecanoate). There is a possible link between Testomet and liver cancer and Andriol can produce nausea if taken in large doses.

Proviron (mesterolone) is another brand of oral androgen but many men find it as ineffective as a placebo.

All in all, oral androgens often prove to be unsatisfactory in their effect and a significant proportion of men with severe testosterone deficiency complain that oral testosterone is not effective. It may not be wise to use oral androgens as an introductory trial in a middle-aged man who has a subtle androgen deficiency, and who is wondering whether male hormone replacement therapy holds the key to wellbeing. If oral androgens are ineffectual, a negative value judgement against all other forms of male HRT may be made, with further attempts being rejected.

Androgen Injections

If a man is considering a short-term trial of male HRT there is probably no more definitive way of proving or disproving its benefit than with a three to four month course of monthly injections of androgen. If a deficiency of testosterone is responsible for the mental, physical and sexual fatigue of middle-age, then the androgen injection should greatly reduce, if not abolish these symptoms within one to two weeks. This brings a great sense of relief and apart from the alleviation of symptoms, the androgen injections can produce a feeling of great energy, vitality and can be a superb anti-depressant.

Suitable androgen injections are Primoteston Depot (testosterone oenanthate) or Sustanon (testosterone propionate), which can be given as a deep oily intramuscular injection into the buttocks each month for three to four months. A follow-up appointment with the doctor should be made two months after the final injection, by which time their effect would no longer be apparent. During this consultation, a decision to abandon or continue with testosterone replacement therapy in the long term can be made. If a patient decides to continue with testosterone replacement for several years or decades, the most effective way in which to deliver the testosterone to the tissues would be through a hormone implant.

Androgen Implants

Each implant contains 200mg of testosterone and if three of these are inserted at once, they will provide good blood levels of testosterone for six months. The implants are buried into the fat of the abdominal wall or buttocks. Most men find these implants very effective and free of side effects. This is understandable as the testosterone is absorbed from the implant directly into the blood, bypassing the liver and carried to the receptive tissues and organs (see Diagram 8, Page 67).

Side Effects Of Androgen Replacement Therapy

If testosterone is given in any form, be it tablets, injections or implants on a long-term basis, it needs to be carefully supervised by a doctor. Testosterone replacement therapy given over several to many years may cause problems and the tablet forms are probably more likely to do this than are the other forms. Ideally, the lowest dose of testosterone should be used to maintain a good quality of mental, physical and sexual wellbeing.

Your partner should be made aware that testosterone replacement therapy can increase the size of the prostate gland. The prostate gland is situated at the neck of the bladder and secretes fluid to add to the sperm during ejaculation. If it becomes enlarged, difficulties may be experienced during the passage of urine with such symptoms as difficulty in beginning urination, dribbling after passing urine, slowness and delay in completing urination and urinary frequency occurring. If these problems persist, surgical removal of the prostate gland may be required. Long-term testosterone replacement therapy may also increase the risk of cancer of the prostate gland. If testosterone doses are excessive, they may produce an unfavourable influence on blood cholesterol patterns thus increasing the risk of cardiovascular disease. Excessive doses may also produce an abnormally high level of red blood cells (polycythaemia).

Overall, testosterone replacement therapy is safe and can be of tremendous value provided it is given by an expert in the field and followed up by annual checkups from a urologist.

Can The Male Menopause Cause Impotence?

Minor degrees of testosterone deficiency do not cause impotence and the level of testosterone deficiency would need to be marked before inability to achieve erection and orgasm occurred. Most men presenting to the doctor with impotence at the time of midlife do not have a significant testosterone deficiency.

Other factors such as general fitness, cardiovascular status, long-term abuse of cigarettes and alcohol, various medications, stress and loss of confidence are more likely to cause impotence especially if these factors occur in combination. Most impotent men have a functional disorder of the "spongy" or erectile tissue in the penis. This erectile tissue is called the corpus cavernosum and during a normal erection it becomes congested with blood. In impotent men this congestion does not occur and so the penis remains small and soft. New treatments available for this problem are vasoactive drugs (Prostin, Prostaglandin E, Alprostadil) that can be self-injected into the erectile tissue of the penis when required. These injections enable the male to regain control of his erections even though he is using artificial means and most users of this method are very satisfied. If this fails, penile implants can be successful. The reader who wishes to know more about male impotence is referred to an excellent and comprehensive book entitled, *It's Up To You* written by Warwick Williams, published by Williams & Wilkins, Adis Pty Ltd.

Female Hormones For Men

It used to be thought that the prime female hormone oestrogen exerted its effects only upon female sexual organs such as the vagina, uterus and breasts. We now know that oestrogen exerts profound and widespread effects upon many other tissues, such as the brain, liver, bones, joints, skin, heart and arteries. In particular, oestrogen has a very favourable effect on blood cholesterol as it helps the enzymes that break down cholesterol and thus reduces the chances of our blood vessels becoming blocked with fatty hard plaques of cholesterol. In the long term, oestrogen helps to reduce diseases of the heart and blood vessels.

This observation has led some of our modern-day scientists to come up with the hypothesis that if we give natural oestrogen to males we can reduce their current high rate of cardiovascular disease. Indeed, there are now clinical trials under way to see if giving natural oestrogen to males between the ages of 30 and 60 will reduce their cholesterol levels and rate of a heart attacks. Oestrogen may also reduce the rate of cancer of the prostate gland so that there could be several ways whereby oestrogen could give men an extra ten years or so of life.

All is not roses, however, as oestrogen being a potent female hormone is likely to exert some possible undesirable side effects in our virile male species. These could be breast tenderness, loss of sex drive, impotence and reduced sperm production.

Nutritional Strategies For The Male Menopause

Diet and lifestyle are supremely important for the male finding himself with reduced mental and sexual performance during midlife.

Exercise is vitally important but I believe, given our current high rate of male cardiovascular disease, that all men should undergo a cardiac stress test (exercise ECG) before initiating an increase in their exercise programme. A good age to have a cardiac stress test is 50 years, or even at 40 years if there is a poor family history.

Some specific nutritional supplements can be tried and these offer a useful alternative to those men who do not feel comfortable about Hormone Replacement Therapy.

NATURAL MALE MENOPAUSE KIT

SUPPLEMENT	DOSE	ROLE
Vitamin E	500 iu daily	Antioxidant action, protects cell structure and reduces oxidative damage to lining of blood vessels. Increases efficiency of oxygen utilisation by cardiac muscle.
Minerals Zinc Selenium Manganese	100 mg daily 50 mcg daily 5 mg daily	Catalysts for enzyme systems thereby increasing metabolic efficiency. Antioxidant action.
Ginseng	500 mg, 3 times daily	Ancient 'glandular tonic' used by Chinese and Russian civilisations.
Hi B Complex tablet	1 daily	Necessary for efficient function of central and peripheral nervous system. Excellent if under stress/alcohol excess.

TABLE 15

MALE MIDLIFE CRISIS

Technically, we know that men cannot go through a literal menopause. However, for many men the phase of midlife brings significant hormonal changes and important physical and psychological changes. Put these all together in a melting pot and you may very well have the ingredients for a male midlife crisis. This is undoubtedly one of the reasons why divorce rates soar at this time and many women get the shock of their lives. These women are left in the well known "empty nest syndrome" with hubby fleeing the familiar domestic scene. Conversely, the male not infrequently gets the "nesting syndrome" and spreads his wings with a younger woman finding that her youthfulness rekindles his feelings of manliness and passion and he feels that life is beginning all over again.

This situation is very emotive and can be extremely traumatic in the short and long term. It could probably be averted in many cases if males received more information and supportive counselling especially with their wives at this time in their lives. In some cases, the timely use of testosterone replacement therapy, even if only on a temporary basis, can bring back the sparkle into a long-term sexual relationship.

If older men keep running off with younger women, what will the women they leave behind do? Well, one obvious strategy is that these women can also get the "nesting syndrome" and run off with younger men! I see quite a few older women doing this and find it an interesting sociological phenomenon. Anyway, there are statistics to support such behaviour, as menopausal women who take natural oestrogen have been found, on average, to live nine to ten years longer than their male counterparts. To avoid loneliness in old age a man ten years younger could probably fit the bill very nicely!

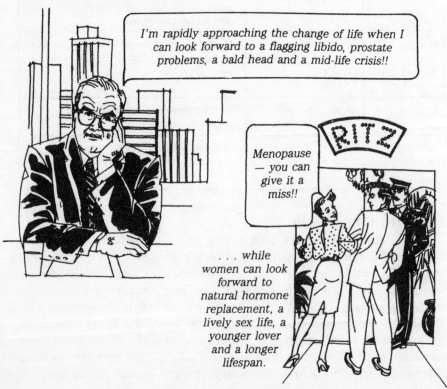

IN SUMMARY — A FAREWELL MESSAGE FROM THE AUTHOR

When you arrive at the menopause there is no reason to fear a change of life for the worse. If you are well informed and aware of all your options you have the tools to maintain and even improve your previous quality and enjoyment of life.

The menopause is a time of learning, self reappraisal and an opportunity to take advantage of the powerful benefits of preventative and nutritional medicine, natural hormone replacement therapy and an anti-ageing plan.

It is a time when you can take control of your life, shaping its destiny and above all take pleasure in being a woman in your own unique style. It is an age when you can have confidence in yourself and your decisions which will give you the persistence to obtain the best care and treatment available today. Whatever you choose, be it ''designer HRT'', orthodox medicine, nutritional medicine, mother nature, or a combination of these, you will be able to overcome your menopausal problems with a positive attitude.

There may be rough patches as you feel and see deep changes evolving in yourself and in these times I hope that this handbook can serve you as a strong and meaningful lifeline. Remember that I am feeling and understanding these changes with you, as are all your sisters on this planet and that if we can gain inspiration, hope and love from each other, that something very precious has been achieved.

I have written this book because you and other women have inspired and taught me so much and I know that we can continue to inspire each other for many years.

I hope this book helps you to enjoy the menopausal years and beyond, and, as far as I can see, the menopause can be fun!

POEM FOR MENOPAUSE
I have some lines on my face from my years of life
They tell me of years in the sun
of sorrows and joys
They tell me of time.....
They tell me I am still alive
They can't be erased
They can be softened....
Do I long to be the smooth-skinned,
freckle-faced kid I once was?
No. I long for the same thing today
that I longed for then:
To be the best I am able to be.

MENOPAUSE

For the attention of the reader:
Your views and comments are important to
the publisher.
The Women's Health Advisory Service
(W.H.A.S.) hopes that you have enjoyed and
profited from this book. We would
appreciate any suggestion that you have
concerning this book which may assist us
and the author to update further
publication. Please send your comments to
the WHAS, 155 Eagle Creek Rd, Werombi, 2570

GLOSSARY

ACNE ROSACEA An eruption of the skin on the face characterised by red inflamed lumps

ADIPOSE TISSUE Fatty tissue

ADRENAL GLANDS Two small glands situated on top of the kidneys which secrete various hormones such as adrenalin, cortisone and sex hormones

AGORAPHOBIA Fear of open spaces

ANABOLIC STEROIDS Synthetic male hormones which stimulate the growth of bone and muscle

ANTIOXIDANTS Substances such as Vitamins A, E and C which protect the cellular structures against oxidative damage.

ATROPHY Wasting or thinning of tissues or organs

AUTO-IMMUNE DISEASES A group of diseases produced by an imbalance in the immune system, whereby the immune system attacks and inflames various tissues of the body.

CANCER A malignant growth/tumour with rapid multiplication of abnormal cells that may spread to and invade distant body parts.

CANCER CHEMOTHERAPY Chemical drugs used to kill cancer cells.

CARDIOVASCULAR DISEASE Diseases of the system of the blood circulation comprising the heart and blood vessels.

CHOLESTEROL A constituent of all animal fats and oils. High blood cholesterol levels increase the risk of cardiovascular disease.

CIRCULATION The recurrent movement of the blood through the various blood vessels of the body.

COLLAGEN A fibrous protein giving elasticity and strength to the skin, bone, cartilage and connective tissue.

CURETTAGE The procedure of surgically scraping a body cavity (such as the uterus) to remove tissue, blood or abnormal growths.

DEFICIENCY Lack of or insufficiency

DOWAGER'S HUMP A forward facing curve on the upper spine, below the neck due to compression of the spinal vertebrae.

ENDOCRINE SYSTEM The network of ductless glands that manufacture and secrete hormones into the bloodstream affecting the function of distant organs and tissues.

ENDOCRINOLOGY The study and treatment of disorders of the glands and the hormones they secrete.

ENDOMETRIOSIS The presence of endometrium (which is normally confined inside the uterine cavity), outside of the uterus, scattered about inside the abdomen and pelvic cavities.

ENDOMETRIAL ABLATION Destruction of the inner lining of the uterus with radio waves or laser beams.

ENDOMETRIUM The mucous membrane forming the inner layer or lining of the uterus.

ENZYMES Proteins which catalyse or facilitate chemical reactions in cells. They are necessary to break down or metabolise drugs and hormones.

EPIDEMIOLOGIST Specialist dealing with the spread of epidemic diseases amongst populations.

ESSENTIAL FATTY ACIDS Fatty acids necessary for cellular metabolism which cannot be produced by the body, but must be supplied in the diet. Suitable sources are oil of Evening Primrose, fish, fish oil, various seeds and nuts.

FALLOPIAN TUBES The small tubes connected to each side of the uterus in which fertilisation of the egg occurs.

FIBROIDS Non cancerous growths of the uterus consisting of muscle and fibrous tissue.

FOLLICLE STIMULATING HORMONE (FSH) A hormone secreted by the pituitary gland which acts on the ovary to stimulate the development of eggs (follicles). These follicles produce oestrogen.

FRIGIDITY (SEXUAL) Sexually unresponsive.

GENETIC ENGINEERING Man-made alteration of the genetic structure of cells for breeding to eradicate diseases or enable cells to synthesize chemicals or hormones.

GLANDS See under endocrine.

HEREDITARY Characteristics or diseases passing through the genes from parents to their offspring.

HORMONE Chemicals produced by various glands which are then transported in the blood to affect distant cells and organs.

HORMONE REPLACEMENT THERAPY (HRT) The administration of hormonal preparations (natural or synthetic) to replace the loss of natural hormone production by various glands.

HYPERTENSION Excessive blood pressure.

HYPOTHALAMUS A major control centre of the brain, regulating temperature, appetite, thirst and the hormonal glands. It is situated at the base of the brain and is directly connected to the pituitary gland.

HYSTERECTOMY Surgical removal of the uterus.

IMPLANT A chemical substance or object that is surgicallly implanted into a part of the body.

INCONTINENCE Inability to restrain or control natural discharges or evacuations such as urine or faeces.

GLOSSARY

INFLAMMATION A condition characterised by swelling, redness, heat and pain in any tissue as a result of trauma, irritation, infection or imbalances in immune function.

INSOMNIA Inability to sleep.

IN-VITRO FERTILISATION (IVF) Fertilisation of the egg by the sperm outside of the body, in a laboratory environment.

LIBIDO Sexual desire.

MENOPAUSE The final cessation of menstruation. The last period.

MENSTRUATION The cyclic (usually monthly) discharge of blood from the non-pregnant uterus. Is also called a menstrual period.

METABOLIC Chemical processes utilising the raw materials of nutrients, oxygen and vitamins along with enzymes to produce energy for bodily functions.

MUCOUS MEMBRANE Lubricating membrane lining an internal surface or an organ such as the gut or genito-urinary canals.

NATUROPATHIC MEDICINE The treatment of illness with naturally occurring substances such as juices, vitamins , minerals, herbs, etc.

OESTRADIOL A natural oestrogen found in the blood. It is the most potent of all the natural oestrogens.

OESTROGEN Female sex hormone secreted by the ovary being responsible for the female physical characteristics of breasts, feminine curves and menstruation.

OESTROGEN RECEPTORS Physical structures on the cell membranes that bind oestrogen.

OESTRONE A natural oestrogen found in the blood.

OSTEOPOROSIS Loss of bone mass due to loss of calcium. Skeletal atrophy. Porous condition of bone.

OVARIES The female sex glands (gonads) located on each side of the uterus which produce eggs and the female sex hormones (oestrogen and progesterone) and a smaller amount of male sex hormones.

PALPITATIONS Irregular or rapid heartbeats.

PAP SMEAR A test in which cells are gently scraped from the cervix and smeared onto a glass slide for examination under a microscope. It is a screening test for cancer of the cervix.

PARATHYROID HORMONE Hormone secreted by the parathyroid glands which controls calcium balance and metabolism.

PEAK BONE MASS The ultimate or maximum amount of bone in the skeleton. Is achieved around the age of 30 years.

PELVIC FLOOR MUSCLES Muscles forming the anatomical floor of the pelvic cavity and giving support to pelvic organs such as uterus, bladder and rectum.

PHARMACOLOGY   The science of drugs and their chemical structure, uses, beneficial and adverse effects.

PITUITARY GLAND   A mushroom shape gland connected by a stalk to the base of the brain. It manufactures many different hormones which in turn control other glands such as the thyroid, adrenal and ovaries.

PLETHORIC ACCUMULATIONS   Congestion with blood.

POST-MENOPAUSE   The period of time after the menopause.

PRE-MENOPAUSE   The years, generally 4-5, immediately before the arrival of the menopause, characterised by a time of hormonal imbalance.

PROGESTAGEN   Synthetic progesterone capable of producing regular menstrual bleeding.

PROGESTERONE   Female sex hormone secreted by the corpus luteum of the ovary.

PROLAPSE   Dropping or protrusion — most often of the rectum (bowel), bladder, uterus or vagina.

RECOMMENDED DAILY ALLOWANCE (RDA)   The daily intake recommended by government health authorities which guarantees an adequate amount of nutrients in normal circumstances. It does not cover all situations such as illness or stress.

SEX HORMONE BINDING GLOBULIN (SHBG)   A protein in the blood that binds and transports the sex hormones oestrogen, progesterone and testosterone. When bound to SHBG the sex hormones are inactive.

STROKE   Brain damage resulting from a disturbance of blood supply to the brain.

TESTOSTERONE   The major male hormone.

THROMBOSIS   A blood clot formed during life in a blood vessel.

TUBAL LIGATION   Surgical sterilisation where the Fallopian tubes are cut and tied or crushed with plastic rings or clips.

UTERUS   Womb.

VAGINA   The genital canal from the uterus to the vulva.

VERTEBRAE   The bone segments forming the spinal column.

VITAMINS   A group of food factors essential for cellular metabolism and maintenance of life.

VULVA   Female external genitalia.

APPENDIX
PRODUCT AVAILABILITY CHART

PRODUCT	SOURCE AND FURTHER INFORMATION
Antioxidant Tablets	Chemist, health food stores, Menopause Support Group
Calcitonin	Your local doctor or endocrinologist
Collagen and Elastin Cream (Bianca's micronised)	Menopause Support Group
Esten	Local pharmacist or Menopause Support Group
Etidronate	Your local doctor or endocrinologist
Ginkgo Biloba	Local pharmacist or health food store
Hormones — natural or synthetic: Progynova, Ogen, Ovestin, Estigyn, Primogyn, Proluton, Primodian Depot, Provera, Duphaston, Primolut, Microlut, Androcur, Aldactone	Your local doctor, menopause clinics, gynaecologists
Maxepa	Local pharmacist
Micelle A Plus E Liquid Antioxidant	Local pharmacist or Menopause Support Group
Cell Repairer Cream	Menopause Support Group
Naudicelle/Naudicelle plus Epanoil	Local pharmacist, health food store, Menopause Support Group
Proguard Antioxidant	Local pharmacist
Pocket Calorie Counter	Newsagents, pharmacies, Allan Borushek, PO Box 250, West Perth, Western Australia 6005
Retin A Cream	Your local doctor - prescription
Super Naudicelle	Local pharmacist, health food store, Menopause Support Group

**MENOPAUSE SUPPORT GROUP: 155 EAGLE CREEK ROAD
WEROMBI, NSW 2570 PHONE: (046) 531 445**

INDEX

REFERENCES

1. R. W. Smith, W. R. Eyler and R. C. Mellingen, *On the Incidence of Senile Osteoporosis,* Annals of Internal Medicine 52 (1960); 773–76.

2. New England Journal of Medicine, 12 July 1990.

3. R. H. Asch, R. B. Greenblatt, Clinics in Obstets and Gynaec, April 1977, Vol 4, No. 1: 85.

4. *An epidemiological evaluation of the risks and benefits of HRT,* Dr Brian Henderson, excerpts from Australian Menopause Society, Inaugural Scientific Meeting, September 89, Brisbane.

5. *The effects of subcutaneous hormone implants during the climacteric,* Linda Cordoza et al. Dept. Obstets and Gynaec, Dulwich Hospital, London, Maturitas, 5 (1984): 177–184.

6. J. W. Studd et al, *Oestradiol and Testosterone Implants,* British Journal of Obstetrics and Gynaecology 1977; 84: 314–315.

7. Wynn Institute for Metabolic Research, *The Lancet,* 1990. 336: 265–269.

8. *Oestrogen–Progestagen Replacement and Cancer Risk,* R. D. Gambrell Jnr., Hospital Practice 15: 81–100, 1990.

9. Armstrong B. K., *Oestrogen Therapy— Boon or Bane?* Medical Journal of Australia 1988; 148: 213–214.

10. MacLennan A. H., *HRT Regimes for the Menopausal Woman,* Current Therapeutics, March 1993, p43.

11. MacLennan A. H., For the Australian Menopause Society. Consensus Statement. Hormone Replacement Therapy and the Menopause. Medical Journal of Australia 155: 43–44, 1991.

12. Tilyard, M. W., et al (1992) New England Journal of Medicine 326: 357–362.

13. American Journal Clinical Nutrition 40, September 1984.

14. Journal of Steroid Biochemistry 25,(5B), 1986.

15. Buist R., Seminar Report 1991, Australian Council for Responsible Nutrition.

16. Weiss N.S., Ure C.L., Ballard J. H., et al. New England Journal of Medicine 1980; 303: 1195–1198.

17. Stampfer M. J., Colditz G. A., Willett W. C. et al, New England Journal of Medicine 1991; 325: 756–762.

18. Steinberg K. K., Thacker S. B., et al, *JAMA*; 1991: 265: 1985–1990.

RESOURCES

SYDNEY

The Menopause Support Group

Offers membership, support and information for menopausal women via seminars in Sydney and various newsletters such as 'What's News' and the 'Hot Flash Newsletter'. For more information phone (046) 531 445 or write to 155 Eagle Creek Rd, Werombi 2570.

To receive information send a large-sized, self addressed envelope to 155 Eagle Creek Rd, Werombi 2570.

Menopause Clinic

The Royal Hospital for Women, Paddington. Phone: (02) 339 4111.

MELBOURNE

Menopause Clinic

The Royal Women's Hospital, Grafton Street, Carlton.

Phone: (03) 344 2000 or 344 2055.

ADELAIDE

Menopause Clinic

Queen Victoria Hospital, 160 Fullarton Road, Rose Park. Phone: (08) 332 4888.

Woman Care Health Centre

520 Anzac Highway, Glenelg East. Phone: (08) 376 0522.

BRISBANE

Menopause Clinic

The Lillian Cooper Centre, 3/71 Bradley Street, Spring Hill, Brisbane.

Phone: (07) 339 4111.

PERTH

Family Planning Association

70 Rose Street, Northbridge, Perth. Phone: (09) 227 6177.

Menopause Clinic

King Edward Memorial Hospital for Women

Bagot Road, Subiaco. Phone: (09) 340 1355.

HOBART

Family Planning Association

73 Federal Street, North Hobart. Phone: (002) 34 7200.

Menopause Support Group

Hobart Women's Health Centre, 9 Pierce Street, Moonah. Phone: (002) 28 0997.

DARWIN

Menopause Clinic

Family Planning Association, Shop 11, Rapid Creek Shopping Centre, Rapid Creek.

Phone: (089) 48-0144

RESOURCES

USA
Menopause
A Friend Indeed
Box 1710, Champlain NY, 12919-1710 Phone: (514) 843-5730 Fax: (514) 843-5681
Provides info and advice on menopause

Osteoporosis — National Foundation
2100 "M" Street, NW, Suite 602, Washington, DC 20037 Phone: (202) 223-2237

American Heart Association
7320 Greenville Ave, Dallas, TX 75321 Phone: (214) 373-6300

The American College of Obstetrics & Gynaecology
404, 12th Street, SW, Washington, DC 20024-2188

MENOPAUSE

THE BODY SHAPING DIET

Do you diet and lose weight in the wrong places?
Do you wish to improve your body shape?
Is your cellulite out of control?
Are you getting fat but don't know why?
Are you looking for an easy, safe, economical and nutritious diet?
If so, the *Body Shaping Diet* is for you!
There are four different body types—ANDROID, GYNAEOID, LYMPHATIC and THYROID—each has distinct hormonal and metabolic differences. To lose weight efficiently and get back your body shape you must follow a diet that has correct food combinations to match YOUR body type. This is called The Body Shaping Diet.

To order *The Body Shaping Diet* mail this coupon to:

WHAS
155 EAGLE CREEK RD, WEROMBI 2570
AUSTRALIA

Or order by PHONE (046) 531 445
or FAX (046) 531 144 using this completed coupon. You need a valid credit card to order by phone or fax.

Please rush me ―――― copies of The Body Shaping Diet Book at $16.95 each plus $2.00 for postage and handling.

Card my credit card (tick correct card):

BANKCARD ☐   MASTERCARD ☐   VISA ☐

YOUR CREDIT CARD NO: ☐☐☐☐ ☐☐☐☐ ☐☐☐☐ ☐☐☐☐

Card Expiry Date ....

OR find enclosed my cheque/money order payable to WHAS for $

Your name ....

Your address ....

P/C .... Your signature ....

Only Bankcard, Mastercard or Visa is accepted. Please fill in all parts of this coupon, including post code, credit card number and expiry date before signing.

DON'T LET YOUR HORMONES RUIN YOUR LIFE

The book "DON'T LET YOUR HORMONES RUIN YOUR LIFE" will be a life-changing experience for thousands of women and men. This book brings you solutions for ■ PMS (Pre-menstrual Syndrome) ■ Postnatal Depression ■ The MALE Menopause ■ After effects of Tubal Ligation ■ Post-hysterectomy Crises ■ Chronic Migraine and Hormonal Headaches ■ Acne and Facial Hair ■ Balding ■ Flagging Libido and Loss of Sexuality ■ Problems with Body Shape and Weight.

It is full of fascinating case histories, diagrams, cartoons and practical treatment tables incorporating the latest advances and scientific discoveries from Australia and overseas in the fields of hormonal and nutritional medicine. This major book in Women's Health is the self-help guide we have all been waiting for.

✂ . . . .

MAIL THIS COUPON TO: WHAS
155 EAGLE CREEK RD, WEROMBI 2570
AUSTRALIA

Please send _____ copies of this book at $15.95 each, plus $2.00 for postage and handling.

Please charge my credit card (tick correct card):

BANKCARD ☐ MASTERCARD ☐ VISA☐

YOUR CREDIT CARD NO: | | | | | | | | | | | | | | | | | | | |

Card Expiry Date . . . .

or find enclosed my cheque/money order payable to WHAS for $_____

Your signature . . . .

Your name . . . .

Your address . . . .

. . . . P/C . . . . Your telephone no . . . .

OR ORDER BY FAX OR TELEPHONE

Telephone: (046) 531 445 to place a credit card order — Bankcard, Mastercard or Visa only accepted.

Fax: (046) 531 144 — fax this completed coupon with your credit card number and personal details filled in.

PERSON YOU WISH BOOK TO BE SENT TO:

To whom (name) . . . .

Address . . . .

. . . . P/C . . . .

Please fill in all parts of this coupon, including post codes, and check your credit card number and expiry date before signing. Prompt delivery in a padded bag is assured.

WOMEN'S HEALTH ADVISORY SERVICE MAIL ORDER

The Women's Health Advisory Service can supply you with nutritional supplements, naturopathic tablets and top quality cosmetics at reasonable prices. All our products are free of artificial chemicals and manufactured to the highest standards. We aim to help women in their search for optimum health and quality of life as they turn away from harsh chemical medicine towards more natural solutions.

To receive our order form, simply fill out the coupon below and post it back to us OR telephone us right now for quicker delivery. Send coupon to:

WHAS
155 Eagle Creek Road
Werombi, NSW 2570

Please send me_____ copies of the WHAS Order Form.
I enclose a large self-addressed, stamped envelope with this coupon.

Your name ....

Your address ....

.... Postcode ....

OR TELEPHONE US ON: (046) 531 445

OR FAX US ON: (046) 531 144

WE CAN MAIL OUR PRODUCTS ALL OVER AUSTRALIA

WOMEN'S HEALTH NETWORK APPLICATION FORM

Do you want to stay in touch with the latest advances in menopause, hormone replacement therapy, anti-ageing techniques, breast care, skin care, nutrition, naturopathic medicine, hormonal problems, improving your sex drive, candida, weight control, body shaping, where to find the best medical specialists and other health issues of vital concern to women? ... **If so**, join our Network! You can write or call our Hotline for this information on (046) 53 1445.

Do you want to receive our exciting Newsletter called *What's News*, published and mailed to you every 8 weeks? The Newsletter contains feature articles on women's health, a Problem Clinic where Dr Sandra Cabot answers common health queries, a skin care section written by our resident beautician, Blanca, and answers from our own resident 'Dorothy Dix', Suzannah Merecia. Articles by gynaecologist Oskar Horky, herbalist Deborah Cooper, and by Trixie Whitmore who writes on how to protect yourself from environmental toxins ... **If so**, join our Network!

Do you want to receive the highest quality natural vitamins, evening primrose oil, skin care products and health books, mailed to you at discount prices? ... **If so**, join our Network!

You can join our Network for 12 months and have all these benefits for only $40.00! What's more, you'll have the opportunity to enter our COMPETITIONS.

HOW TO JOIN THE WOMEN'S HEALTH ADVISORY NETWORK

Send $40.00 to Women's Health Advisory Service (WHAS) with your details and you will be entered on our Computer Mailing List and receive a Membership Card and number, your first Newsletter, a Naturopathic Table and 1 **FREE** bottle of Evening Primrose Oil. Send your $40.00 to WHAS, 155 Eagle Creek Road, Werombi 2570.

If you have a credit card (Visa, Mastercard or Bankcard), you can phone us on (046) 53 1445 or fax on (046) 53 1144 with your details.

Your name ....

Your address ....

.... Postcode ....

Your phone ....

Send Cheque/Money order for $40.00 to WHAS or DEBIT my Credit Card

Visa ☐   Mastercard ☐   Bankcard ☐

Credit card no. ☐☐☐☐☐☐☐☐☐☐☐☐☐☐☐☐

Card expiry date .... Your signature ....